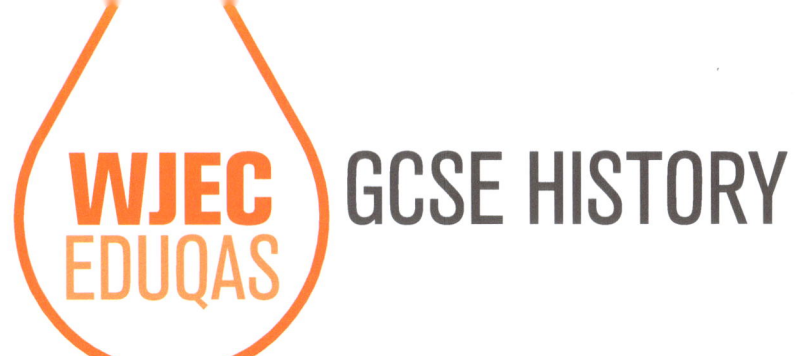

CHANGES IN HEALTH AND MEDICINE IN BRITAIN

c.500 to the present day

R. Paul Evans • Alf Wilkinson

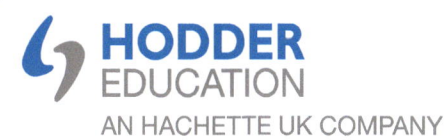

Every effort has been made to trace all copyright holders, but if any have been inadvertently overlooked, the Publishers will be pleased to make the necessary arrangements at the first opportunity.

Although every effort has been made to ensure that website addresses are correct at time of going to press, Hodder Education cannot be held responsible for the content of any website mentioned in this book. It is sometimes possible to find a relocated web page by typing in the address of the home page for a website in the URL window of your browser.

Orders: please contact Hachette UK Distribution, Hely Hutchinson Centre, Milton Road, Didcot, Oxfordshire, OX11 7HH. Telephone: +44 (0)1235 827827. Email education@hachette.co.uk Lines are open from 9 a.m. to 5 p.m., Monday to Friday. You can also order through our website: www.hoddereducation.co.uk

ISBN: 978 1 4718 6817 7

© R. Paul Evans, Alf Wilkinson 2016

First published in 2016 by
Hodder Education,
An Hachette UK Company
Carmelite House
50 Victoria Embankment
London EC4Y 0DZ

www.hoddereducation.co.uk

The authorised representative in the EEA is Hachette Ireland, 8 Castlecourt Centre, Dublin 15, D15 XTP3, Ireland (email: info@hbgi.ie)

Impression number   10 9

Year   2024

All rights reserved. Apart from any use permitted under UK copyright law, no part of this publication may be reproduced or transmitted in any form or by any means, electronic or mechanical, including photocopying and recording, or held within any information storage and retrieval system, without permission in writing from the publisher or under licence from the Copyright Licensing Agency Limited. Further details of such licences (for reprographic reproduction) may be obtained from the Copyright Licensing Agency Limited, www.cla.co.uk.

Cover photo © WellcomeLibrary

Illustrations by Barking Dog Art and Tony Randell

Typeset in India by Aptara Inc.

Printed and bound by CPI Group (UK) Ltd, Croydon CR0 4YY

A catalogue record for this title is available from the British Library.

CONTENTS

Introduction 4

The Big Story: changes in health and medicine in
Britain, c.500 to the present day 7

Chapter 1	Causes of illness and disease	14
Chapter 2	Attempts to prevent illness and disease	30
Chapter 3	Attempts to treat and cure illness and disease	42
Chapter 4	Advances in medical knowledge	54
Chapter 5	Developments in patient care	64
Chapter 6	Developments in public health and welfare over time	80

Historic environment studies

Chapter 7	The village of Eyam during the Great Plague of 1665–66	94
Chapter 8	The British sector of the Western Front, 1914–18 and the treatment and care of the wounded	107

Examination Guidance 121

Glossary 132

Index 134

Acknowlegements 136

Introduction

About the Eduqas course

During this course you must study **two** components (each carrying a weighting of 50 per cent):

Component One: Studies in Depth

This is in two parts and consists of:
- A British Depth Study
- A non-British Depth Study

Component Two: Studies in Breadth

This is in two parts and consists of:
- A Period Study
- A Thematic Study, which includes the study of a historical site.

These studies are assessed through four examination papers:

Component One consists of a two-hour examination split into two papers – one hour on the British Depth Study and one hour on the non-British Depth Study.

Each study is assessed by compulsory questions focusing on the analysis and evaluation of historical sources and interpretations. There are also questions testing second order historical concepts such as continuity, change, consequence, significance, similarity and difference.

Component Two consists of a two-hour examination split into two papers – 45 minutes on the Period Study and one hour 15 minutes on the Thematic Study.

Each study is answered by five compulsory questions on the Period Study paper and seven compulsory questions on the Thematic Study paper. The main focus is on second order historical concepts but there is also some testing of source analysis and evaluation skills.

About the book

This book covers the Option 2F Changes in health and medicine in Britain, *c*.500 to the present day, which is a thematic study and is part of Component Two. The book is divided into eight chapters.

1. Causes of illness and disease

This chapter examines the key question: *What have been the causes of illnesses and disease over time?* It examines the problems which faced medieval society, such as poverty, famine, warfare and poor hygiene, with reference to the Black Death of the fourteenth century, together with the Great Plague of the seventeenth century. The effects of industrialisation and the incidence of typhoid in the nineteenth century is explored, as well the spread of bacterial and viral diseases in the twentieth century.

2. Attempts to prevent illness and disease

This chapter focuses on the key question: *How effective were attempts to prevent illness and disease over time?* It examines the early methods of prevention particularly in relation to the Black Death; the use of alchemy, soothsayers and medieval doctors. The application of science to help prevent disease in the late eighteenth and early nineteenth centuries is explored. The work of Edward Jenner in relation to inoculation and vaccination is examined, along with the discovery of antibiotics and developments in the field of bacteriology.

3. Attempts to treat and cure illness and disease

This chapter focuses on the key question: *How have attempts to treat illness and disease changed over time?* It examines the treatments and remedies used during the medieval era such as herbal medicine, barber surgeons and the use of leeches. It explores the development of antiseptics by Joseph Lister and anaesthetics by James Simpson. Changes during the twentieth century are also explored, such as the development of radiation by Marie Curie; the roles of Fleming, Florey and Chain in developing antibiotics; Bernard and transplant surgery; and modern advances in cancer treatments and surgery. Alternative treatments are also examined.

4. Advances in medical knowledge

This chapter focuses on the key question: *How much progress has been made in medical knowledge over time?* It examines medical ideas during medieval times including the influence of alchemy, astrology and the theory of the four humours. The medical work of Vesalius, Pare and Harvey is explored, together with the advances in medical knowledge through the work of Pasteur and Koch. Advances during the twentieth century including developments in scanning techniques, the discovery of DNA and genetic research are also explored.

5. Developments in patient care

This chapter focuses on the key question: *How has the care of patients improved over time?* It examines the role of the church and monasteries in delivering patient care up to the mid-sixteenth century, followed by the development of voluntary charities and endowed hospitals during the seventeenth and eighteenth centuries. The influence of Florence Nightingale in the development of professional nursing during the late nineteenth century is examined, together with the influence of Liberal reforms upon patient care during the early twentieth century. The major changes resulting from the Beveridge Report and the creation of the NHS are examined.

6. Developments in public health and welfare

This chapter focuses on the key question: *How effective were attempts to improve public health and welfare over time?* It examines public health and hygiene in medieval society, followed by developments in the sixteenth and seventeenth centuries. The impact of industrialisation on public health in the nineteenth century is explored through the work of Edwin Chadwick and Victorian attempts to improve public health. Efforts to improve housing and pollution in the twentieth century are also explored.

7. Study of a historic environment: the village of Eyam during the Great Plague of 1665–66

This chapter focuses on the significance of the impact of the Great Plague upon the village of Eyam during the 1660s and how this contributed to changes in health and medicine. It examines the arrival of the plague at Eyam in 1665, the symptoms of the disease, the effectiveness of the cures and remedies available to the villagers, as well as the impact of the death toll. The setting up of a quarantine zone and its effectiveness are examined, together with the significance of events at Eyam in changing attitudes towards the prevention of disease.

8. Study of a historic environment: the British sector of the Western Fronts of 1914–18 and the treatment and care of the wounded

This chapter focuses on the significance of the impact of new weapons and methods of warfare upon the treatment and care of the wounded men fighting in the trenches and how this contributed to developments and changes in health and medicine. It examines the nature of fighting on the Western Front; the impact new battle strategies and new weapons had on the nature and type of wounds; and injuries received by soldiers fighting in the trenches. The processing and treating of casualties, new developments in surgical methods and medical advances such as blood transfusions, plastic surgery and the use of radiography are examined. The significance of these new treatments and care of the wounded on the Western Front for changes in health and medicine is assessed.

Eduqas Examination

COMPONENT TWO: Studies in Breadth

A Thematic Study

2F: Changes in health and medicine in Britain, *c*.500 to the present day.

Time allowed: 1 hour 15 minutes

1. Use Sources A, B and C to identify one similarity and one difference in the care of patients over time. **[4 marks]**

2. Which of the two sources is the more reliable to a historian studying developments in public health over time. **[6 marks]**

3. Describe the development of surgery during the nineteenth century. **[5 marks]**

4. Explain why developments in germ theory were important in the prevention of illness and disease in the nineteenth and twentieth centuries. **[9 marks]**

5. Outline how attempts to prevent illness and disease have changed from *c*.500 to the present day. **[16 marks and 4 marks for SPaG]**

6(a). Describe two attempts to stop the spread of the Great Plague in Eyam in 1665. **[8 marks]**

6(b). Explain why the environment of Eyam during the Great Plague was significant in changing attitudes towards the spread of disease in the seventeenth century. **[12 marks]**

Total marks for the paper: 64

In Question 1 you have to pick out information from the three sources to identify both similarities and differences.

In Question 2 you have to analyse and evaluate the reliability of both sources. You should make reference to the content, the authors and the nature and purpose of each source. You should provide a judgement upon which of the two sources is most reliable and why you think this.

In Question 3 you have to demonstrate your own knowledge and understanding of a key feature. You should aim to include specific factual detail.

In Question 4 you have to identify a number of reasons to explain why a key development/issue was important or significant. You should aim to include specific factual detail.

In Question 5 you need to use your own knowledge to provide a detailed, well-structured account, explaining how and why the key issue named in the question has changed/developed over time. Remember to take care with spelling, punctuation and grammar.

In Question 6(a) you have to demonstrate your knowledge and understanding of a key feature. You should aim to include specific detail and cover a number of points.

In Question 6(b) you have to identify reasons why the historical site you have studied was significant in influencing changes and developments in health and medicine. You will need to justify your reasons with good factual support.

How this book will help you with WJEC Eduqas History

It will help you to learn the content

Is your main worry when you prepare for an exam that you won't know enough to answer the questions? Many people feel that way – particularly when a course covers over 1000 years of history! And it is true, you will need good knowledge of the main events and the detail to do well in this thematic study. This book will help you acquire both the overview and the detail.

The author text explains the key content clearly. It helps you understand each period and each topic, and the themes that connect the topics. Diagrams also help you to visualise and remember topics. Drawing your own diagrams is an even better way to learn!

The book is full of sources. This course deals with some big issues and sources help pin those issues down. History is at its best when you can see what real people said, did, wrote, sang, watched, laughed about or cried over. Sources can really help you understand the story better and remember it because they help you to see the big concepts and ideas in terms of what they meant to people at the time.

Think questions direct you to the things you should be noticing or thinking about in the sources and text. They also help you practise the kind of analytical skills that you need to improve in history.

The **Topic Summary** at the end of every chapter condenses all the content into a few points, which should help you to get your bearings in even the most complicated content. You could read that summary before you even start the topic to know where you are heading.

It will help you to apply what you learn

The second big aim of this book is to help you apply what you learn, which means to help you think deeply about the content, develop your own judgements about the themes, and make sure you can support those judgements with evidence and relevant knowledge. This is not an easy task. You will not suddenly develop this skill. You need to practise studying an issue, deciding what you think and then selecting from all that you know the points that are really relevant to your argument. One of the most important skills in history is the ability to select, organise and deploy (use) knowledge to answer a particular question.

The main way we help you with this is through the **Focus Tasks**. These are the big tasks that appear at the end of each chapter so that you can build your big picture of the story of medicine and health over time. We then ask you to revisit the focus task at the end of the chapter to help you think through the big issues.

It will help you prepare for your examination

If you read all the text and tackle all the Focus Tasks in this book you should be well prepared for the challenges of the exam, but to help you more specifically:

- **Practice questions** at the end of each chapter provide exam-style questions.
- **Examination guidance** appears on pages 121–31. These pages take you step by step through how best to approach and answer the types of exam questions. They provide some sample answers that help you to see what an effective answer might look like.

The Big Story: changes in health and medicine in Britain, c.500 to the present

This thematic unit covers a vast period of time – over 1500 years – and includes a lot of detail. Each chapter covers the continuing story of the development of health and medicine in Britain. You will need to keep on connecting these little stories to the big story. That is what this section helps you with. It gives you an overview of the themes you will be studying and some activities to help you see the patterns over time. Good luck!

Feeling poorly

What happens today when you feel unwell? Where do you go to get help? Perhaps you self-diagnose. You go either to the supermarket or the pharmacy and buy medicine, or perhaps ask the pharmacist's advice. How do you know the medicine you buy is safe to use? How do you know it will work? You've probably seen the adverts on the television or in the newspaper, but how do you really know it is safe to take and to use? Who controls the development and marketing of medicines today? Who do you think did it in medieval times? Did they even have medicine in medieval times?

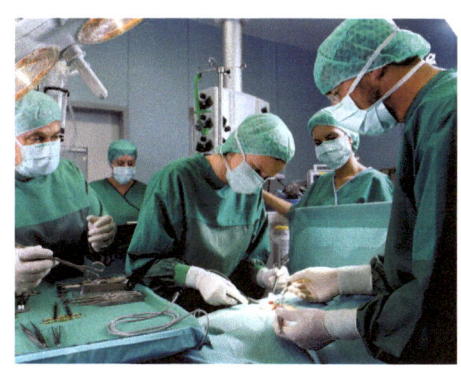

You might visit an 'alternative medicine' provider. Some people prefer 'natural healing', using herbs and traditional methods, such as Chinese acupuncture, homeopathy or osteopathy. More and more people are convinced the best way to diagnose illness and then cure it is through natural remedies.

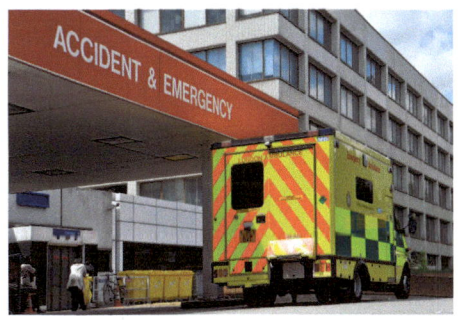

If it is an emergency you might go straight to the accident and emergency (A&E) department of your local hospital, or call an ambulance to take you there. You might have a bit of a wait but there is emergency treatment available 24/7, with nursing staff and hospital consultants on call to deal with any kind of emergency.

Most likely you will make an appointment with your GP (general practitioner). It is usually possible to get an appointment within a day or so. Once there you might see the doctor, a nurse-practitioner or even the practice nurse. Whoever you see will try to decide what is wrong with you using a variety of techniques. They might take your temperature: when was the thermometer invented? How did they take your temperature before thermometers? They might listen to your breathing using a stethoscope. How did they do that before stethoscopes were invented? They might ask for a urine sample: this is widely used to test for some illnesses. Or take a blood test. Perhaps they might just look at you, or listen to what you have to say. If they can decide what is wrong with you they might issue a prescription for medicine and send you on your way.

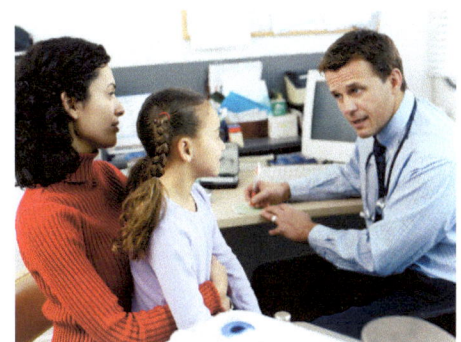

But what if they cannot decide? What happens then? In all probability you will be referred to a specialist, and there will be yet more tests. Eye tests, MRI scans, physio tests; specialists have a huge array of tests to probe and try to discover the cause of your ill health. It might be a quick process, but sometimes it takes a long time to finally discover the *cause* of your illness.

Thinking about health and medicine

> **ACTIVITY**
>
> Below you can see some of the events that help us to tell the story of health and medicine over the last 3000 years or so. Can you put these events in the appropriate place on the timeline?
>
> 1. Draw your own version of the timeline below and pencil in each of the events in the appropriate place.
> 2. You will find the correct dates for each of these events on the bottom of page 10. Plot the correct dates onto your timeline.
> 3. Do you find any of these answers surprising? If so, why?
> 4. What does your timeline tell us about health and the people?
>
> You will be coming back to this timeline after you have finished the topic and will then have the opportunity to amend your thinking.

EVENT A: TREATMENTS – PENICILLIN, THE FIRST ANTIBIOTIC

'We had an enormous number of wounded with infections, terrible burn cases among the crews of armoured cars. The usual medicines had absolutely no effect. The last thing I tried was penicillin. The first man was a young man called Newton. He had been in bed for six months with fractures of both legs. His sheets were soaked with pus. Normally he would have died in a short time. I gave three injections of penicillin a day and studied the effects under a microscope. The thing seemed like a miracle. In ten days' time the leg was cured and in a month's time the young fellow was back on his feet. I had enough penicillin for ten cases. Nine were complete cures.'

EVENT B: TREATMENTS – HERBAL MEDICINE

'Medicine for dimness of the eyes: take the juice of the celandine plant, mix with bumblebees' honey, put in a brass container then warm until it is cooked and apply to the eyes.'

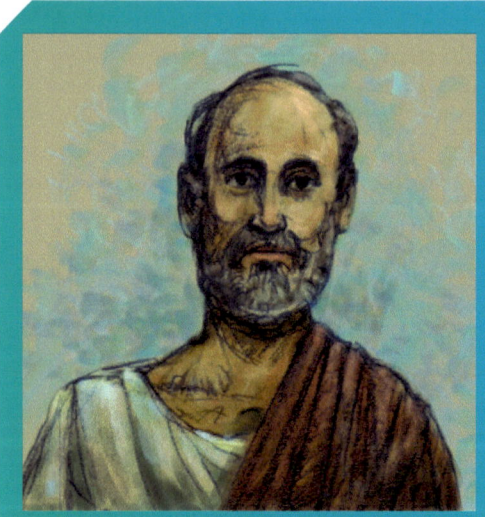

EVENT C: EXPLAINING DISEASE – THE FOUR HUMOURS

Hippocrates wrote: 'Man's body contains Four Humours – blood, phlegm, yellow bile and melancholy (black) bile. When all these humours are truly balanced, he feels the most perfect health. Illness occurs when there is too much or too little of one of these humours or one is entirely thrown out of the body.'

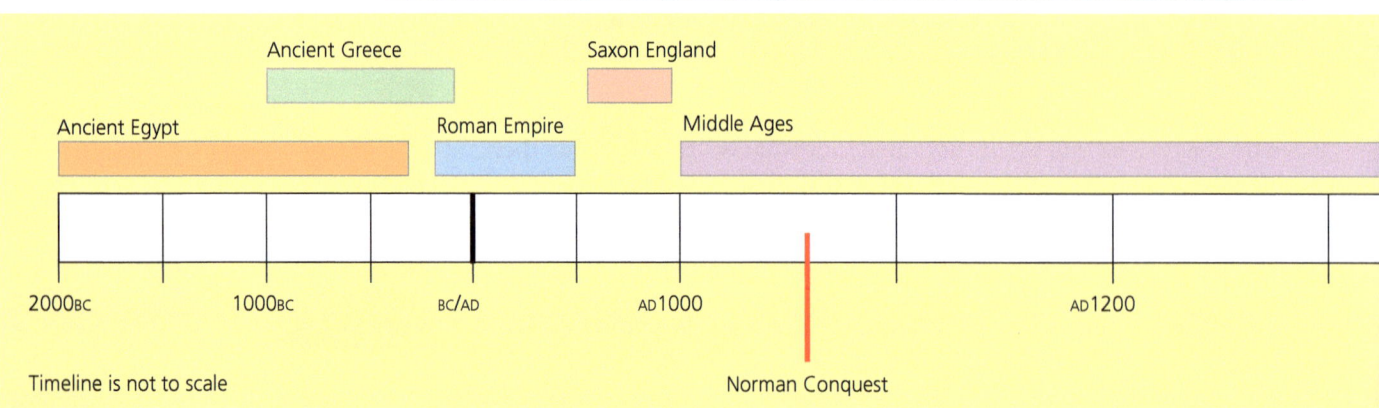

Timeline is not to scale

EVENT D: EXPLAINING DISEASE – GOD SENDS DISEASE

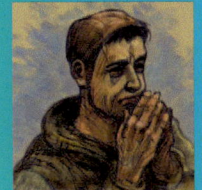

'Terrible is God towards men. He sends plagues of disease and uses them to terrify and torment men and drive out their sins. That is why the realm of England is struck by plagues – because of the sins of the people.'

EVENT E: PUBLIC HEALTH – THE NHS BEGINS

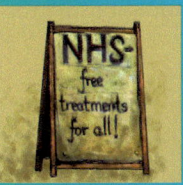

'On the first day of free treatment on the NHS, Mother went and got tested for new glasses. Then she went further down the road to the **chiropodist** and had her feet done. Then she went back to the doctor's because she'd been having trouble with her ears and the doctor said he would fix her up with a hearing aid.'

EVENT F: EXPLAINING DISEASE – PASTEUR AND GERM THEORY

Louis Pasteur, a French scientist, published his 'germ theory' suggesting that bacteria or 'germs' were the true causes of diseases. His germ theory replaced all previous ideas about the causes of disease.

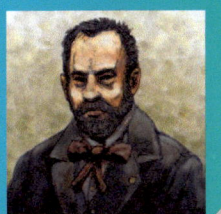

EVENT G: TREATMENTS – THE BLACK CAT REMEDY

'The stye on my right eyelid was still swollen and inflamed very much. It is commonly said that rubbing the eyelid with the tail of a black cat will do it much good so, having a black cat, a little before dinner I tried it and very soon after dinner the swelling on my eyelid was much reduced and almost free of pain.'

EVENT H: TREATMENTS – WASH, EXERCISE, DIET

'Every day wash face and eyes with the purest water and clean the teeth using fine peppermint powder. Begin the day with a walk. Long walks between meals clear out the body, prepare it for receiving food and give it more power for digesting.'

EVENT I: SURGERY – WITHOUT ANAESTHETICS

Robert Liston, a famous London surgeon, once amputated a man's leg in two and a half minutes but worked so fast he accidentally cut off his patient's testicles as well. During another high-speed operation Liston amputated the fingers of his assistant and slashed the coat of a spectator who, fearing he had been stabbed, dropped dead with fright. Both the assistant and the patient then died of infection caught during the operation or on the hospital ward. Liston worked really fast because there were no **anaesthetics**.

EVENT J: PUBLIC HEALTH – FRESH WATER, BATHS AND SEWERS

Sextus Julius Frontinus wrote: 'There was a great increase in the number of reservoirs, fountains and water-basins. As a result the air is purer. Water is now carried through the city to **latrines**, baths and houses.'

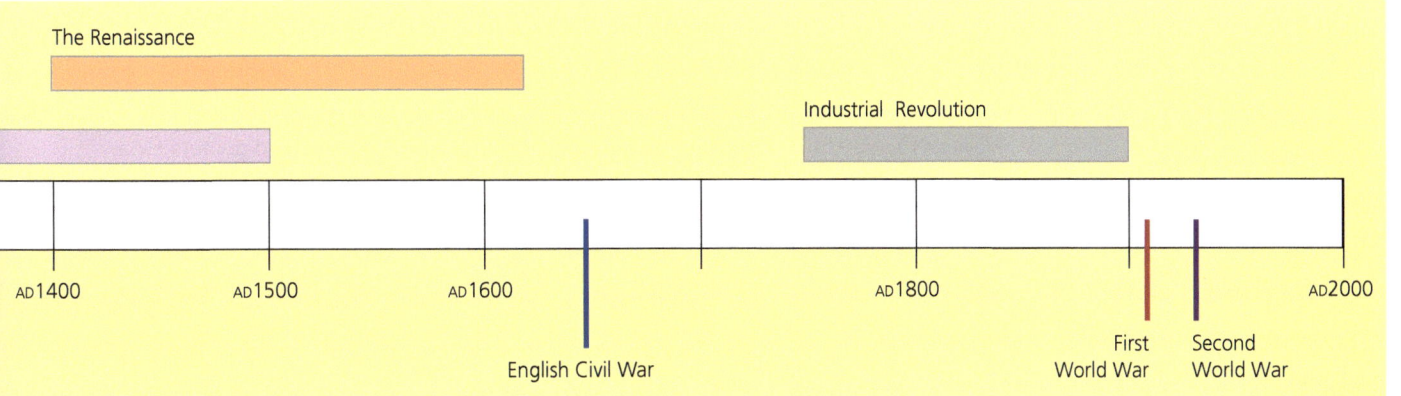

Treating sick people

Deciding what is wrong with you is only half the battle, however. How do you put it right? What *cure* should the doctor use to put right any illness? There are plenty of potential cures to choose from. Whole industries have grown up producing medicines, tablets and technology to treat patients, and to make money out of it. How is the doctor or specialist to decide which is the best treatment to use? What works for one person might not work for another. And how do they decide the right level of dose in each particular case? In other words, how do they get the 'cure' right?

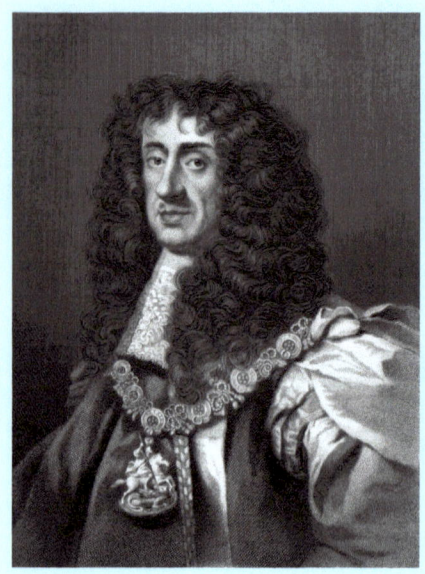

Feeling poorly in the seventeenth century

In early 1685 Charles II felt poorly. He called in his doctors. According to some accounts there were 14 of them, who were often arguing over cause and potential cure. These were, of course, supposed to be the best doctors in the country! On 2 February Charles fainted, so the doctors had to decide what to do with him. First of all they bled him, taking over 400 ml of blood from his right arm. He did not respond, so they took another 200 ml of blood, and gave him an emetic, to make him vomit. This was a mixture of antimony, sacred bitters, rock salt, mallow leaves, violet, beetroot, camomile flowers, fennel seed, linseed, cinnamon, cardamom seed, saffron, cochineal and aloes. This would in theory clear any impurities out of his system. The next day they took more blood (300 ml this time), and gave him a mixture of barley water and syrup to gargle. He was also given more laxatives to clear out his bowels. His treatment seemed to consist of continuous bloodletting, laxatives and emetics. Not surprisingly he became weaker and weaker. He did not respond to the treatments and on the morning of 6 February Charles II died.

Recent research suggests that King Charles II died of kidney failure, probably linked to gout. Gout was a common disease among the upper classes at the time. The very worst treatment for kidney failure is to bleed a patient, so it appears that King Charles' doctors played a large part in killing him! So why did they bleed him? What were they trying to do? Were doctors in the seventeenth century so ignorant that they did not know the cause of the illnesses they were being asked to treat? Is the situation any different today? Today's doctors still find it hard to pinpoint the cause of some illnesses, and to effectively treat them.

ACTIVITY: MEDICINE MINI-DICTIONARY

As you work your way through this book you will come across various herbs, medicines, diseases or operations that you may not have heard of before. When you do, carry out your own research to find out all about them. Write your own definition of each one, with notes, and create your own mini-dictionary of medicine through time.

THINK

1. Do you think King Charles' doctors knew the *cause* of his illness? Do you think they had a clear idea of how to *cure* the illness?
2. How similar, and how different, are the ways in which Charles' doctors and doctors today approach someone who is poorly?
3. In your opinion, has the way sickness is treated improved, or got worse, between 1685 and today? Explain your answer.

Answers to the activity from pages 8–9:
A 1943 B 900s C 450BC D 1348 E 1948 F 1860 G 1788 H 390 BC I 1830s J 100

But people are healthier now, right?

You would think that people are healthier in today's world. People eat better, more regular meals, have higher incomes, there is much more food available, everyone is well-housed and warm, people are educated into making healthy choices. Surely that means they are healthier today. But it seems not everyone agrees.

> **Human Teeth Healthier in the Stone Age Than Today**
>
> (*Health Magazine*, 19 February 2013)

> Medieval diets were far more healthy. If they managed to survive plague and pestilence, medieval humans may have enjoyed healthier lifestyles than their descendants today.
>
> (BBC News website, 18 December 2007)

> The UK is among the worst in western Europe for levels of overweight and obese people. In the UK, 67% of men and 57% of women are either overweight or obese. More than a quarter of children are also overweight or obese – 26% of boys and 29% of girls.
>
> (*Guardian*, 29 May 2014)

The stories above cast doubt on the idea of people being healthier today than ever before. The story from *Health Magazine* is based on archaeological examination of teeth. They found evidence of fewer cavities, less oral disease and less bone disorder than today. The BBC News website story is based on research into medieval records carried out by a Shropshire GP. The *Guardian* news story is taken from NHS England statistics. Can it really be the case that people today are less healthy than in medieval times? How can we investigate this idea further? How might you measure if people are healthier now than in previous periods of history?

One measure might be how long people live – if people live longer today then surely that means they are healthier?

The evidence is pretty clear from this data. Men, on average, now live twice as long as they did in Anglo-Saxon times. Surely that tells us that men, at least, are healthier today than 1000 years ago? But do our ideas change if we use another set of statistical data?

THINK

1. What are the strengths of figures such as those showing the average age of death?
2. What are the limitations of these kinds of figures? Remember, until recently infant mortality was so high (often 33 per cent of children failed to reach the age of seven) that *average* figures for life expectancy are lowered.
3. According to the data in the table, when were British men healthiest? How can you tell?
4. According to this data, when were British men unhealthiest? How can you tell?
5. How tall do you think, on average, British men will be in:
   a) 2100
   b) 2200
   c) 2500?

Period	Average male height
Anglo Saxons	5 feet 6 inches (168 cm)
Normans	5 feet 8 inches (173 cm)
Medieval	5 feet 8 inches (173 cm)
C17th	5 feet 5 inches (165 cm)
Victorians	5 feet 5 inches (165 cm)
C20th	5 feet 8 inches (168 cm)
Today	5 feet 10 inches (178 cm)

▲ Table: Average height of British males, compiled from various sources, but mostly skeletal data

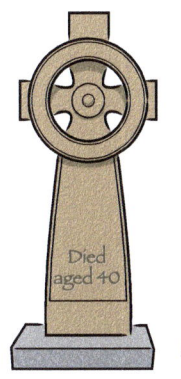
Anglo-Saxon

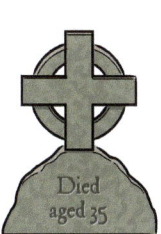
Medieval

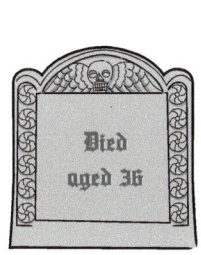
Seventeenth century

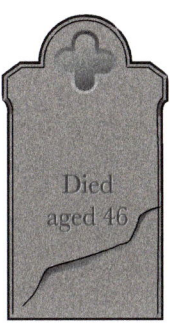
Victorians

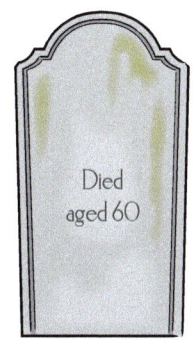
1930s

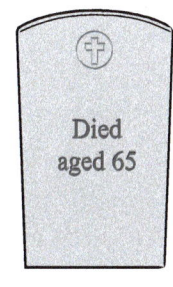
1950s

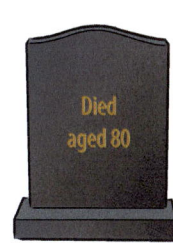
Today

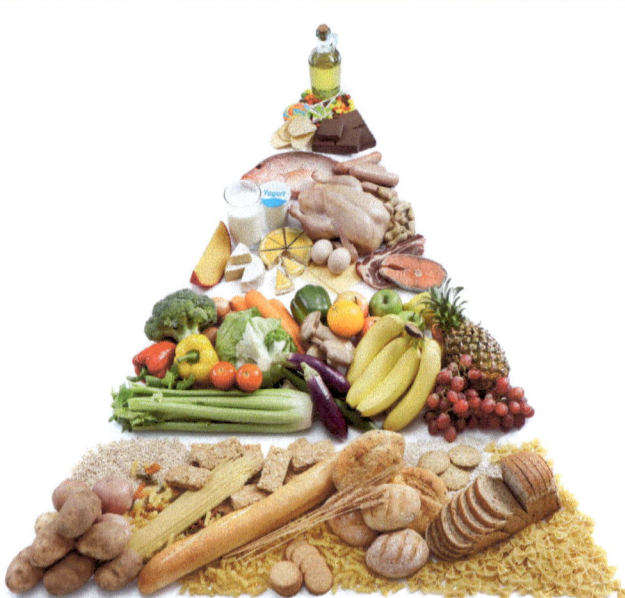

▲ **Source A:** A healthy living pyramid from the Australian government showing the proportions of different food groups in a healthy diet

> **THINK**
> 1. Can you think of any other measures we might use to decide whether or not people are healthier today than in previous centuries?
> 2. Find out what you would eat if you were to follow the 'Stone Age Diet'.
> 3. Why, if people are healthier than ever before, do they need all this advice?
> 4. Why are modern people so obese?
> 5. What are the foods we eat that are bad for us? And who decides what is good and bad?

Making sense of all this data

People are living longer, and growing taller, at least according to the data shown here. Does that mean we are healthier? The figures on the previous page refer solely to men, and are averages. These figures therefore are only part of the picture. (There is much less skeletal data for women, for example, hence there is not enough reliable information to compile a 'height' list for women covering the period we are studying.) Leaving aside the limitations of the data, we are faced with a series of conflicting evidence; some suggesting people are now healthier, but equally some suggesting people may live longer but are not necessarily healthier. How can we reconcile this conundrum, and begin to reach a conclusion?

It is very easy to get data for today, or from the last two centuries. Since Victorian times the government has collected masses of data about every aspect of people's lives. But how do you find meaningful data from the seventeenth century, or the thirteenth century? Would it perhaps be more helpful if we looked at child mortality, or deaths in childbirth, both of which have been major killers throughout much of history? What other aspects of peoples' lives might we consider?

Nowadays people are bombarded with advice on how to live a more healthy life: drink less alcohol, give up smoking, take more exercise, eat less sugar and fats, and so on. Nearly every week it seems new advice appears to help people deal with their unhealthy lifestyle choices. New diets are continually proposed. One of the latest is the 'Stone Age diet', where you eat and exercise like Stone-Age hunter-gatherers.

ACTIVITIES

1. On your own version of the table below, keep your own 'food diary' for a week. Make a note of what you eat and when.

	Monday	Tuesday	Wednesday	Thursday	Friday	Saturday	Sunday
Breakfast food							
Breakfast drinks							
Lunch food							
Lunch drinks							
Dinner food							
Dinner drinks							
Snacks							

2. Study the 'healthy living pyramid' from Source A. Use a different colour for each section of the pyramid, and then highlight your food diary to show how much food you are eating from each of the different groups.
3. Now use the pyramid to decide whether or not you are eating healthily.
4. If you are eating unhealthily, make a list of how you could change your diet to make it healthier.

Keeping clean

You have already discovered, from your timeline activity (see pags 8–9) that the Ancient Greeks clearly knew of the link between cleanliness and healthiness. So why was it so difficult to keep clean throughout most of history?

The answer is much the same as the reason most people drank ale or 'small beer' instead of water – not because they were addicted to alcohol but that water was both expensive and very dirty! It was quite common for waste to be discharged into a river before drinking water was taken out of the same river. There were few laws and health regulations. Local corporations (councils) and mayors were reluctant to take action to provide clean water because it would cost money, and, as most people were relatively poor, it would be the small number of richer people who would have to foot the bill. People had to collect their water from wherever they could. And that often meant the local river or stream. What is surprising is the lengths people went to in order to try to keep themselves and their houses clean. Some towns had public baths from the early 1500s and, of course, if you were rich you could have your own private water supply brought direct to your house.

Everyone today gets treated the same, don't they?

If you are ill then under the National Health Service (NHS) everyone has equal access to care, at least in theory. Whether you are rich or poor, live in the town or the countryside, are young or old you get treated by the NHS. However, consider this newspaper headline, from January 2015, highlighting the inequalities in cancer care. Apparently in deprived areas patients sometimes get poorer treatment than in richer areas.

> **National Audit Report highlights gap between rich and poor which could prevent 20,000 deaths per year**
>
> (*Daily Mirror*, 15 January 2015)

Was this the case in the past? Did everyone get the appropriate treatment whether they could pay for it or not? We have already seen that King Charles II was treated very differently to any patient today, and he presumably had plenty of money to pay for medical attention.

How successful might your treatment be?

Most doctors today would be very surprised if their 'cures' for various illnesses did not work. It might take a while to find the correct dose, or the right medicine, but usually, in most cases, patients recover. Some illnesses are more deadly than others. Some cancer recovery rates are still very low, for example. But other illnesses that were fatal in times gone by, like measles, have all but been eradicated.

> **Source B:** Killer diseases of late twentieth-century Britain
> - Cancer
> - Heart disease
> - Respiratory disease (for example, flu)
> - Liver disease
> - Dementia/Alzheimer's disease
> - Accidents

THINK

1. Why was it so difficult for most people to keep clean throughout most of history?
2. Do you agree that people are healthier today than they were in other periods of history?
3. Study Source B.
   a) Which of these diseases do you think of as 'old people's' diseases?
   b) Which of these diseases do you think of as 'young people's' diseases?
   c) Which do you think of as 'lifestyle' or 'affluence' diseases?
   d) Which do you think were killer diseases in earlier times?

1 Causes of illness and disease

This chapter focuses on the key question: What have been the causes of illness and disease over time?

Not surprisingly, medieval people did not really understand the causes of most diseases. Famine and war were perhaps the main killers of this period. A bad harvest caused by drought or flood, too hot or too cold weather, meant malnourishment for many. And malnourished people catch disease more easily. Dysentery, typhoid, smallpox and measles were all widespread. Some historians estimate that perhaps 10 per cent of England's population in the early fourteenth century died of these diseases. Childbirth was a dangerous time for women, and it is likely that 30 per cent of children died before the age of seven. Poverty was, perhaps, the biggest killer though. This chapter explores how the causes of disease change throughout the period, but also to a surprising extent remain the same.

FOCUS TASK

As you work through this chapter make a 'Cause of illness and disease' card for each cause you come across. On it, make bullet points that show the impact this had. You will need these cards in subsequent chapters. The first one has been done for you.

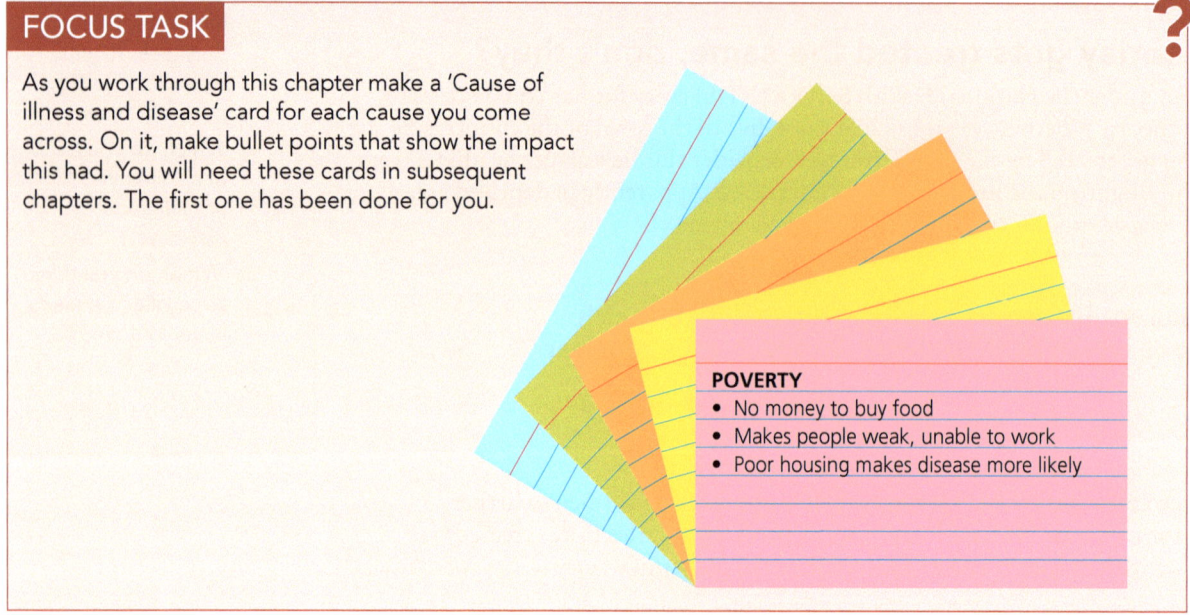

POVERTY
- No money to buy food
- Makes people weak, unable to work
- Poor housing makes disease more likely

Problems in the medieval era – poverty, famine and warfare

Poverty

Most people in medieval England depended on their fields for food. A bad harvest meant hunger or starvation; a good harvest meant plenty to eat and often some to sell to those living in the towns. By 1300 the population of England was around 4.75 million, probably the largest it had ever been. There had been 30 years of good harvests. Most people lived in the countryside and worked in agriculture. Perhaps 25 per cent of rural families had enough land to support themselves, but many did not. Many had no land at all. It is estimated that 40 per cent of rural families had to buy some or all of their food. Often farm work had to be supplemented by wage labour in order to make enough money to survive. As landowners were enclosing more and more land for sheep – much of the country's wealth came from the wool trade – paid work was often hard to come by.

Most people therefore lived on or near the poverty line, eating bread and pottage, a kind of stew made from beans, peas and oats, with herbs or a little meat or fish if available. Rabbit, chicken and fish were sometimes eaten, but the penalties for poaching were severe. A bad harvest meant difficult times for many people. Many animals would be slaughtered in the autumn because of a lack of winter fodder. Child mortality was high and malnutrition common for many, even in a good year.

1 Causes of illness and disease

Famine

Famine was a regular occurrence – sometimes more fatal than others. In 1069, for example, William the Conqueror, angry with continuing Anglo-Saxon rebellions in the north, destroyed a whole swathe of land between the River Humber and the River Tees. His men even ploughed salt into the ground so crops would no longer grow! Thousands died in the resulting famine. Source A below gives details of more famines during the Anglo-Saxon period.

> **Source A:** Extracts from the *Anglo-Saxon Chronicle*, from Terry Jones and Alan Ereira's *Medieval Lives*
>
> AD1082
>
> … and this year also was a great famine.
>
> AD1086
>
> And this year was a very heavy season, and a swinkful and sorrowful year in England, in murrain of cattle, and corn and fruits were at a stand, and so much untowardness in the weather, as a man may not easily think …
>
> AD1087
>
> … Afterwards came, through the awfulness of the weather as before mentioned, so great a famine over all England, that many hundreds of men died a miserable death through hunger … yet such things happen for folk's sins, that they will not love God and righteousness.

There were other famines recorded in 1258, 1437–49 (when peasants in Chester were recorded as resorting to making bread from peas) but perhaps the harshest famine in England, and most of Europe, was in 1315–17 when torrential rain ruined planting and harvesting, not for one year but for three.

> **Source B:** Extract from the *Annales of John de Trokelowe*, a monk at St Albans Abbey
>
> In the year of our Lord 1315, hunger grew in the land … Meat and eggs began to run out, capons and fowls could hardly be found, animals died of pest, swine could not be fed because of the excessive price of fodder. A quarter of wheat [usually on sale for five shillings] or beans or peas sold for twenty shillings, barley for a mark, oats for ten shillings. A quarter of salt was commonly sold for thirty five shillings, which in former times was quite unheard of. The land was so oppressed by want that when the King came to St. Albans on the feast of St. Laurence [10 August] it was hardly possible to find bread on sale to supply his immediate household.

The poor harvest was compounded by the death of animals from disease and a shortage of fodder – the meat could not even be preserved as salt was too expensive for many. Most of the seed grain was eaten so it was impossible to sow enough crops when the weather improved in 1318, so the effects of the famine rumbled on until 1324 or 1325. It is estimated that between 10 and 15 per cent of England's population died during this famine. There are (unconfirmed) reports of cannibalism, and many children were abandoned by parents unable to feed them.

> **THINK**
>
> 1. How useful is Source B in helping us find out about the impact of the famine in 1315?
> 2. What is the difference between the famines of 1082–87 (Source A) and 1315 (Source B)?
> 3. What were the major effects of famine?
> 4. Why were the poor so susceptible to famine?

> **THINK**
>
> 1 Why do you think young people were so at risk of dying from ill-health in medieval times?
> 2 Which of the medieval killer diseases are still dangerous today?
> 3 Was the passage of a medieval army more dangerous for the soldiers, or for the villagers whose land they passed through?
> 4 Study Source C. Why might an illuminated prayer book show someone being hanged?

Medieval warfare

Archaeological excavations of Anglo Saxon (c.450–1066) and Viking (c.800–1066) sites show bodies with unhealed wounds inflicted by sword or axe, often gangrenous. There is a suggestion that an epidemic killed many otherwise healthy males in the Viking army winter camp at Repton in Derbyshire in 873–74. At the start of the medieval period armies were relatively small, and therefore deaths in battle few. Later in the period armies were much bigger. Edward I, King of England from 1272–1307, often called out 10,000 cavalry and 30,000 infantry in his wars with Wales and Scotland. At the Battle of Towton, in 1461, an estimated 22,000 to 28,000 soldiers were killed fighting.

Wars were also dangerous if you were in a besieged town, city or castle. If you held out too long or refused calls to surrender, then once the attacking army broke in inhabitants were often killed or driven off with nothing. In 1224, for example, once Henry III captured Bedford Castle all the remaining defenders were hanged.

Finally, most medieval armies tried to provision themselves as they travelled across the country. Enormous quantities of fodder, grain and food were required. Medieval monarchs could seize whatever they wanted – usually promising to pay later, but many did not – and thus frequently villages, farms, towns were left short of food for themselves. The passage of an army through your neighbourhood could lead to having your house burnt down, your livestock stolen or your crops taken. Medieval soldiers were paid infrequently so were not averse to helping themselves to food!

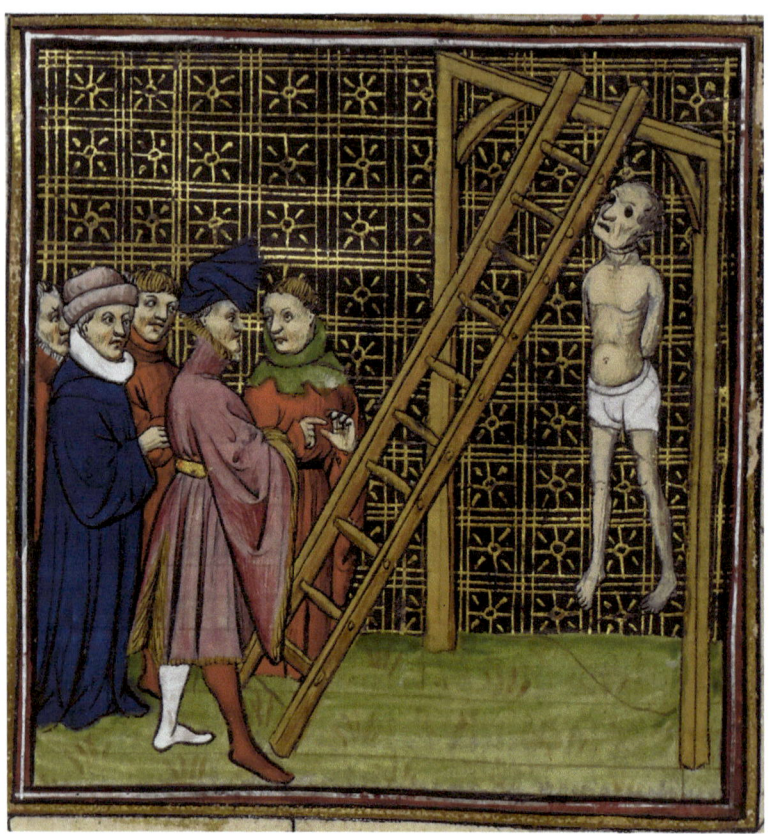

▲ **Source C:** Medieval illuminated letter showing someone being hanged

Accidental death

Accidents were common and often fatal as, for example, the case of Maud Fras, who was killed by a large stone accidentally dropped on her head at Montgomery Castle in Wales in 1288. At Aston, Warwickshire in October 1387, Richard Dousyng fell when a branch of the tree he had climbed broke. He landed on the ground, breaking his back, and died shortly after. Or the case of Johanna Appulton who in August 1389 in Coventry was drawing water when she fell into the well. The incident was witnessed by a servant who ran to her aid and while helping her fell in also. This was overheard by a third person who also went to their aid – he too fell in – and all three subsequently drowned.

Storing crops over winter brought their own problems too. 'Saint Anthony's Disease', for example, was caused by a fungus growing on stored rye in damp conditions. Once the rye was ground into flour and baked into bread those who ate it developed painful rashes and in some cases, even died.

1 Causes of illness and disease

What did medieval people think made them ill?

During this period people had a wide range of beliefs about the causes of illness.

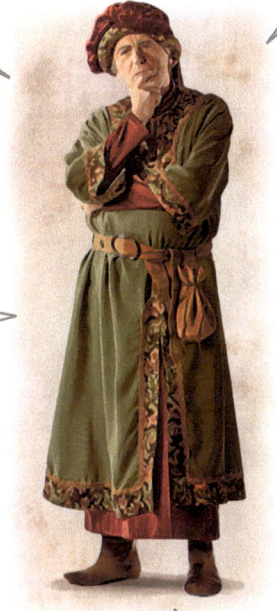

God

Religion played a huge part in most people's lives so it is not surprising that people thought God had a part to play in the spread of diseases. Christian Anglo-Saxons often blamed illness and disease on God, saying he was reminding people of the need to live a decent life. If someone was living a sinful life, then a difficult illness was God's way of punishing them for their sins. And if society as a whole was being sinful, or moving away from the true path of faith and the directions of the pope, then an epidemic or plague was a just reward, sent by God, to remind people of their duties to the church.

Bad smells

Some people began to notice the link between disease and bad air, or bad smells. Mortality was higher in the towns and cities than in the countryside. People lived closer together, alongside their animals and their filth. Travellers often said you could smell a town long before you could see it. So it is hardly surprising that many people thought disease was spread by bad smells infecting neighbours and friends.

Everyday life

Most people believed illness and early death was inevitable. So many children died before the age of seven that in many ways it seemed quite natural. Also childbirth was a very dangerous time for women, and it was expected that if his wife died a man would need to remarry to provide his children with a new mother. Warfare and famine were frequent. Everyday life was an uncertain business.

The supernatural

Mystery and magic and the supernatural world were used by some to explain unexpected happenings. Viking sagas suggest many believed disease was caused by magic, or even elves and spirits. Witchcraft was feared and many believed the world was full of demons trying to cause mischief and death. Any sudden diseases or misfortunes could easily be blamed on the supernatural, especially as the church painted a picture of a life where 'good' fought 'evil'.

The four humours

By far the widest-held belief was that people were ill because their **four humours** were out of balance. Every doctor agreed with Hippocrates and Galen that illness was caused by losing their equilibrium. Every doctor had a chart showing which illnesses were caused by which humour that they would use alongside a zodiac chart showing when was the best time to treat illnesses, plan an operation or even pick the herbs needed for medicine. (See Chapter 4 for more on the four humours and zodiac chart.)

ACTIVITIES

1. Which do you think are the best explanations of the causes of illness outlined on this page? Rank them in order along a line like this one:

   Best explanation ——————————————— Worst explanation

2. Repeat the activity, this time showing which explanations you think medieval people would find most convincing. Can you explain any differences?

Lack of hygiene in the medieval and early modern eras

> **ACTIVITY**
>
> Look carefully at this picture of London in 1347. Some of the things making life unhealthy are highlighted with a text box. Others are not. Make a list of all that you can find.

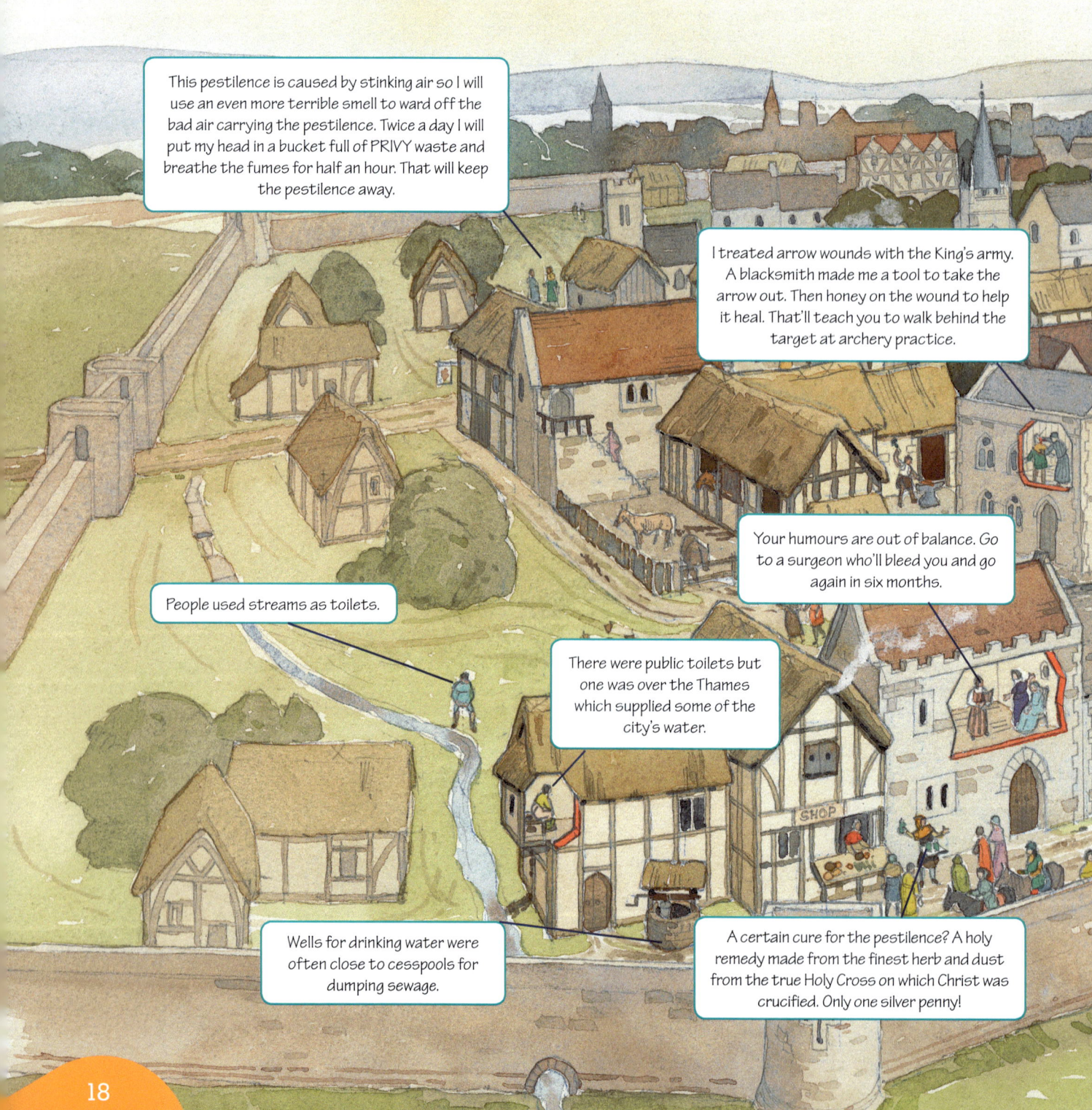

1 Causes of illness and disease

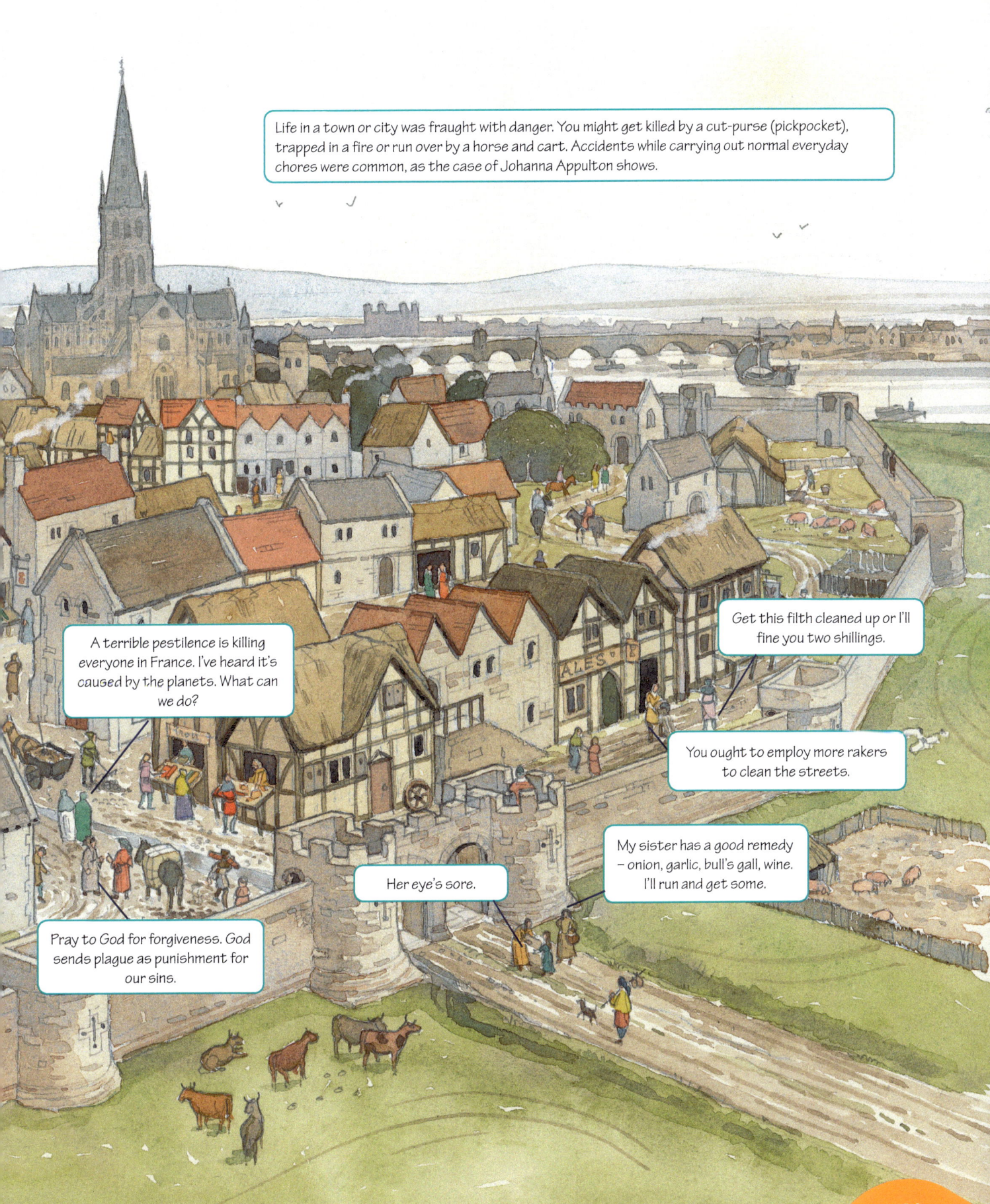

What made towns so unhealthy?

In the Middle Ages towns were much smaller, and fewer in number, than today, yet they were still very unhealthy places. There was little regulation or restriction on what you could or could not build. Houses were crowded together and sanitation very limited. Improvements depended on the corporation that ran the town and most wanted to keep costs as low as possible.

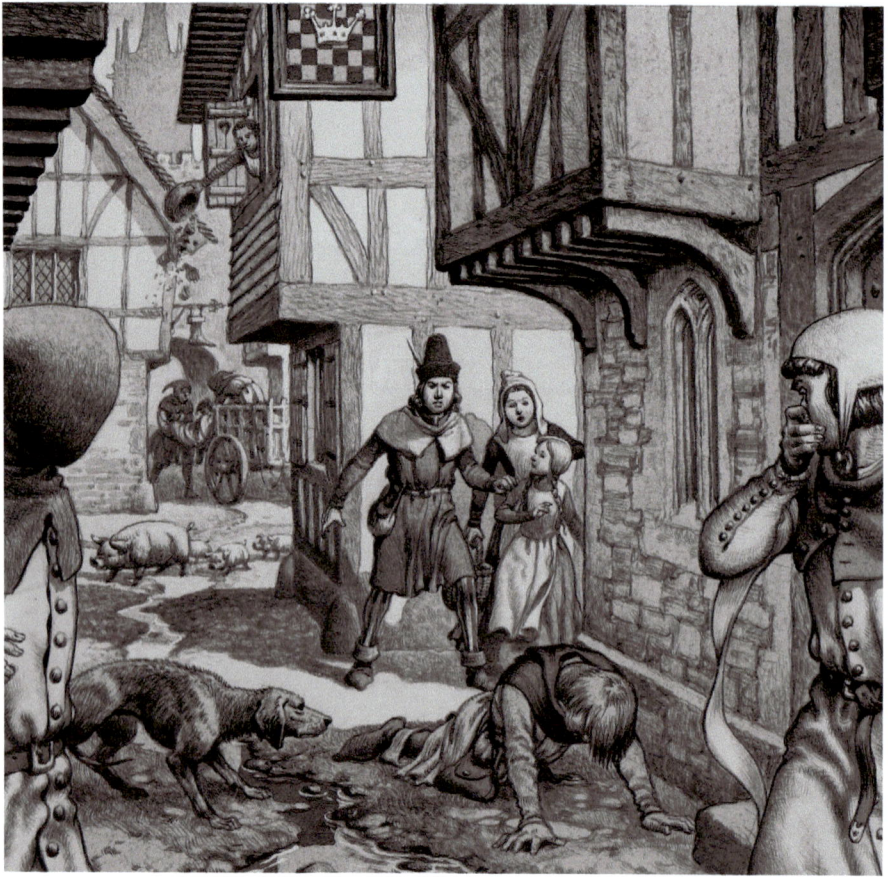

▲ **Source D:** A medieval town, from *Look and Learn* magazine in 1976

Life in a town or city was fraught with danger. You might get killed by a **cut-purse**, or run over by a horse and cart. You might get caught up in a fire. Fires spread rapidly as most houses were made of wood and thatch.

Homes were unhealthy too. Floors were covered in straw or rushes which were rarely changed. This was the perfect breeding ground for rats, mice, lice and fleas – ideal for spreading diseases and infection. There were few windows, and usually smoke from the fire – essential for cooking – would have to make its way out via a hole in the roof. Only rich people had glass windows and chimneys, so homes were dark and smoky; not very healthy!

Towns were unhealthy because so many people lived so close together. There were few regulations about building or waste disposal. Clean water was in short supply, often taken from rivers and streams that were contaminated with waste. Butchers brought their animals into the town or city alive and slaughtered them – they were then faced with the problem of how to get rid of the waste. Industries like tanning were carried on nearby, creating smells and waste. There was no 'zoning' in towns – industry and houses were mixed together higgledy-piggledy. There were no dustbins or dustbin men to collect the rubbish – it just accumulated in the streets until the rain washed it away. Cesspits might be dug next to wells, allowing one to contaminate the other – or the cess pit was emptied infrequently – you had to pay people to take the waste away.

Everywhere there were animals – horses for transport, creating tons of dung every week; or domestic pigs roaming around eating scraps before being slaughtered. There were no sewers, so household waste was chucked out into the street and left to rot. If you were unlucky the overnight piss-pot might be chucked out of an upstairs window as you were passing below. Keeping food fresh was difficult, so you had to shop for food every day, and shopkeepers would try to sell food that was going off rather than throw it away. Water for washing – either clothes or people – was hard to come by, so people were not perhaps as clean as they might be. Water for drinking was also rare, hence most people would drink 'small-beer' rather than risk the water. What was permissible in the countryside or in a small village became deadly in towns. Disease spread quickly. No wonder medical people thought disease was spread by bad smells!

THINK

1. Why, in your opinion, were towns so unhealthy in medieval times?
2. How did this cause illness and disease?
3. Look at Source D. Identify all the health hazards shown in this image. Can you find at least six?
4. To what extent does Source D agree with the text on this page? Which offers the better interpretation of medieval towns – Source D or the text? Why?

1 Causes of illness and disease

A case study of the Black Death: what does this disease tell us about the causes of disease in medieval times?

In 1348 a ship docked at Melcombe in Dorset, bringing with it the Black Death. People must have known it was coming as it had spread across the known world from Asia. Its impact was devastating. In some places whole villages were wiped out. Historians disagree over just how many people were killed by the epidemic of 1348–49, but estimates vary from 50 to 66 per cent of the British population.

What did people think caused the Black Death?

The truth is that people at the time did not really know much at all about the causes of ill-health, but they had plenty of theories! Here are just some of the suggested causes of the Black Death in England.

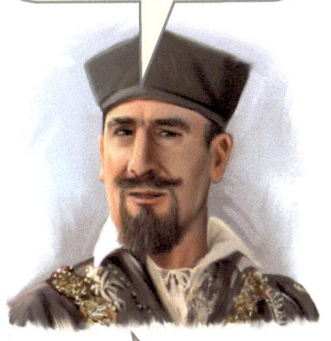

"Bad smells, from an overflowing privy or rotting food, corrupt the air."

"Invisible fumes are spreading across the country."

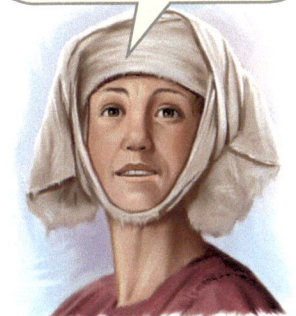

"The four humours are out of balance in each victim."

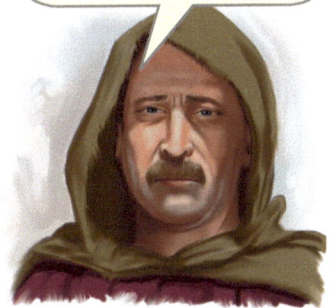

"The planets can explain it. Saturn is in conjunction with Mars and Jupiter and that always means something bad happens."

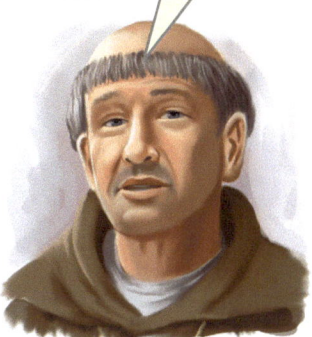

"God is angry with us – not enough people have been going to church or behaving properly."

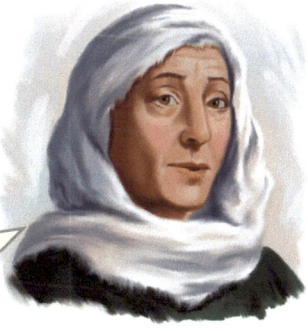

"People have been wearing fancy new clothes, and showing off their wealth. This has made God very angry and therefore he has sent a plague, like he did in biblical times, to teach us to behave better."

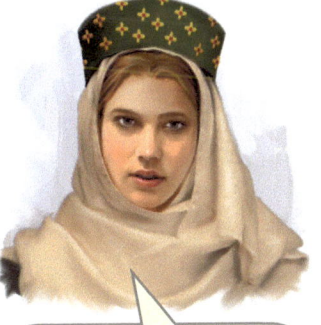

"There was a huge earthquake in China in 1347. China is where the Black Death started in 1347."

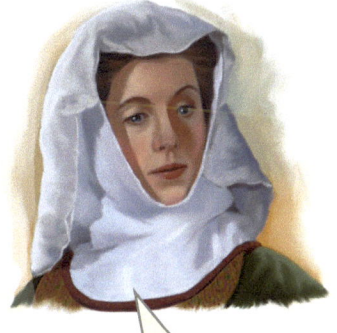

"Jewish people have poisoned the wells and springs."

It is important to remember that historians today still debate the exact causes of the Black Death. The prevailing argument is that it was bubonic plague spread by rats. However, others suggest that it was spread by close contact between humans. Archaeologists have not found lots of rat bones, suggesting the plague wasn't spread by rats, and the fact that mortality rose in winter suggests the Black Death may have been something other than bubonic plague all together. If we find it difficult to understand what caused the disease, what chance did people in the Middle Ages have of understanding the cause of, and then effectively curing, such a rampant disease?

> **THINK**
> Do you find any of these causes surprising? If so, why?

Being ill in the seventeenth century

The biggest killer diseases in the seventeenth century were: 'fever, consumption, teeth, griping in the guts, and convulsions'. Just the very descriptions tell us how little physicians and surgeons understood about the causes of disease, let alone cures. These diseases are not so very different from the killer diseases of the sixteenth or fifteenth centuries, or, for that matter, earlier times.

The Diseases and Casualties this Week.

Disease	Number	Disease	Number
Abortive	2	Imposthume	1
Aged	32	Infants	7
Bleeding	1	Kingsevill	1
Childbed	5	Mouldfallen	1
Chrisoms	9	Kild accidentally with a Carbine, at St. Michael Wood-street	1
Collick	1	Overlaid	1
Consumption	65	Rickets	9
Convulsion	41	Rising of the Lights	2
Cough	5	Rupture	2
Dropsie	43	Scalded in a Brewers Mash, at St. Giles Cripplegate	1
Drowned at S Kathar. Tower	1	Scurvy	4
Feaver	47	Spotted Feaver	2
Flox and Small-pox	15	Stilborn	13
Flux	3	Stopping of the Stomach	11
Found dead in the Street at Stepney	1	Suddenly	1
Griping in the Guts	15	Surfeit	7
		Teeth	27
		Tissick	12
		Ulcer	1
		Vomiting	1
		Winde	1
		Wormes	1

Christned: Males — 121, Females — 111, In all — 232
Buried: Males — 195, Females — 198, In all — 393 Plague — 0
Decreased in the Burials this Week — 69
Parishes clear of the Plague — 130   Parishes Infected — 0

The Assize of Bread set forth by Order of the Lord Maior and Court of Aldermen; A penny Wheaten Loaf to contain Eleven Ounces, and three half-penny White Loaves the like weight.

▲ **Source E:** Weekly mortality bill, London, 21–28 February 1664

THINK

1. Look carefully at the bill of mortality for London, February 1664 (Source E). Which are
   a) the diseases that kill the most people
   b) the diseases that kill the least people?
2. How has this list changed since medieval times?
3. What has happened to the population of London in the week 21–28 February 1664? What does that tell us about how healthy life in London was?
4. Why does the bill of mortality refer to 'the plague'? What was the impact of the plague in that week?

1 Causes of illness and disease

A case study of London in 1665: what does the Plague tell us about changes in the way people thought disease was caused?

Plague came often to major towns and cities. In 1604, 30 per cent of the population of York died in an outbreak of the plague. In 1665 around 100,000 people died of the plague in London. That was nearly 25 per cent of the population. Other towns and cities were affected too, for example Eyam in Derbyshire (see Chapter 7). Most doctors fled, fearing for their lives. Wealthy people fled the city for their country houses until the plague left, but in many cases that just spread the plague to new places. Studying the plague, and what people thought caused it, gives us a great opportunity to decide how much had changed between the Black Death in 1348–49 and the Plague in 1665.

What did people at the time think caused the plague?

The truth is that people in the early modern period did not really know much at all about the causes of the plague, but they had plenty of theories. Below is a picture of a plague doctor wearing the protective outfit designed by Charles de Lorme in Italy in 1619.

> **THINK**
> 1 Look closely at the plague doctor's clothes and equipment in Figure 1.1. What do they tell you about what people at the time thought caused the Plague?
> 2 Look back at page 21 on what people in medieval Britain thought caused the Black Death in 1348.
> 3 From your work in this chapter, which of these causes do you think people in 1665 still believed caused the Plague?

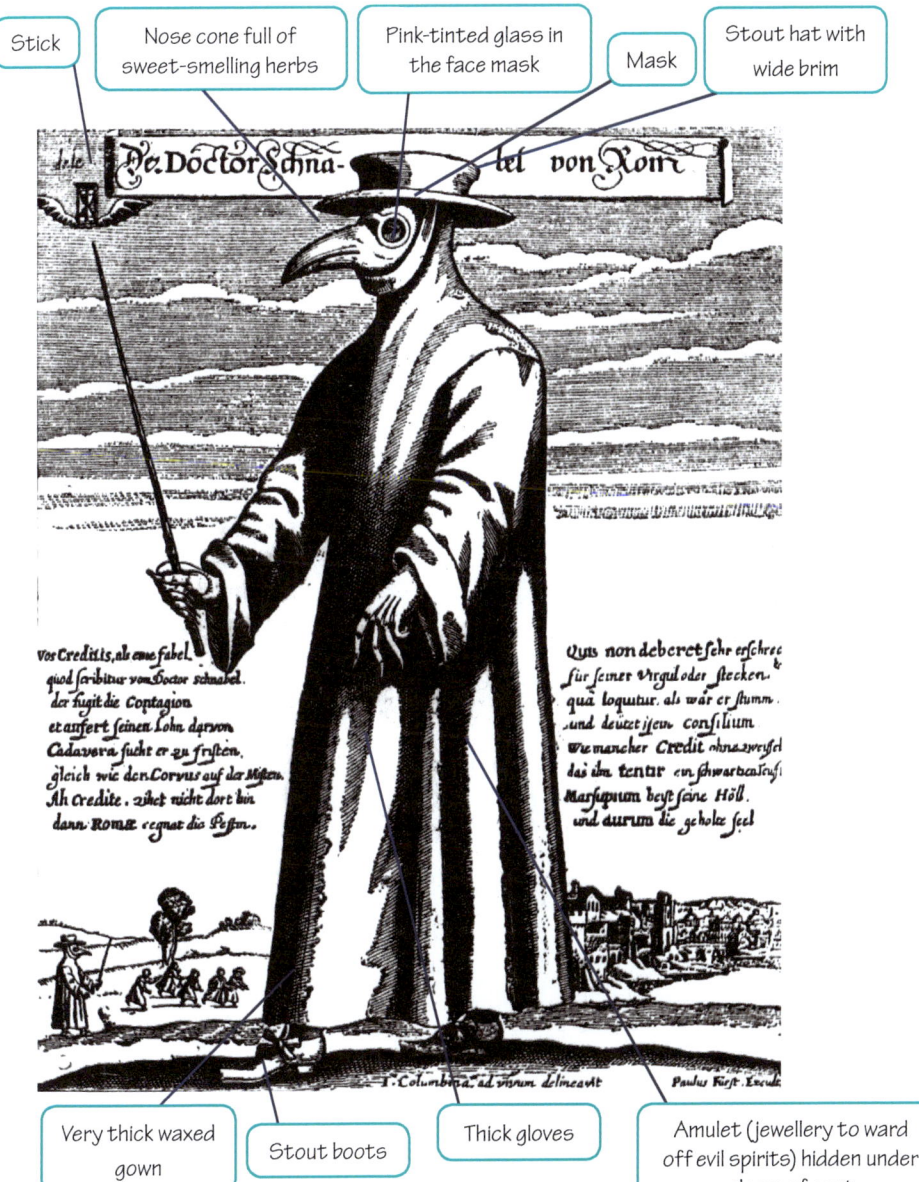

Figure 1.1: A plague doctor wearing a protective outfit designed by Charles de Lorme in Italy in 1619

23

THINK

1. Study Source F. Try to imagine what it would be like living in one of these houses. How do you keep clean and tidy? Where do you get your water from? Where do you go to the toilet? How likely is your washing to dry or to stay clean? What would happen if your neighbour fell ill?
2. To what extent does Doré's engraving agree with the other evidence we have from Victorian times about living in the new towns?
3. What were the 'killer diseases' of the nineteenth century?
4. How did industrial jobs bring new causes of illness and disease?
5. How similar, and how different, were the causes of illness and disease in medieval towns and the new industrial towns?

The effects of industrialisation and the incidence of cholera and typhoid in the nineteenth century

Were the new industrial towns really that bad to live in?

The Victorians were exceptional at collecting data, and this is a great help in trying to discover what life was like in industrial towns. For example, we know that in Bethnal Green, in East London, in 1842 richer people lived on average to the age of 45, whereas labourers lived until they were just 16. In Manchester at the same time 57 per cent of all children died before they reached their fifth birthday. Social surveys from the time show that often a whole family lived in one room, or in a cellar liable to flooding; many children shared a bed, and toilets and water supplies were shared by many families. There are plenty of other statistics we could use but these examples tell us that yes, indeed, the new industrial towns were grim to live in.

Contagious diseases, such as typhoid, typhus, diarrhoea, smallpox, tuberculosis, scarlet fever, whooping cough, measles and chicken pox, all spread rapidly in such poor and overcrowded conditions. No wonder 57 per cent of children died before they reached the age of five. Perhaps the best indicator of how bad conditions were is the prevalence of rickets, known in the nineteenth century as 'the English Disease'. This is a crippling bone disease common in infants caused by calcium deficiency and lack of fresh air and sunlight, and is a clear indicator of malnutrition.

New hazards in industrial life

Added to the overcrowding were the new industrial diseases. Young boys forced to climb up chimneys came into contact with soot and gases. Percivall Pott, an English surgeon, identified scrotal cancer in many of these chimney boys. Young girls making matches at factories across London developed 'phossy-jaw' caused by the fumes from the phosphorous used to make the match heads. Parts of the jaw would be eaten away, or glow greenish-white in the dark. It also caused brain damage. Coal miners developed pneumoconiosis, a disease of the lungs, caused by inhaling dust below ground. Machines in the new textile factories rarely had guards, and hands and arms were often caught in the machines. There were few regulations controlling working conditions and accidents were common, with no compensation and little prospect of further work.

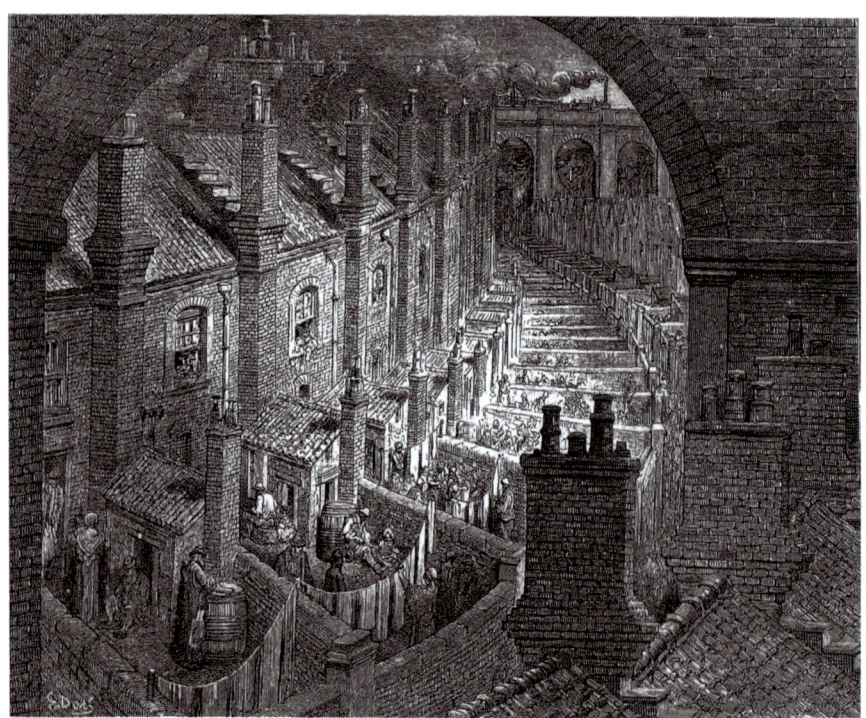

▲ **Source F:** Engraving by Gustave Doré of part of London in 1872

1 Causes of illness and disease

Here comes cholera

Perhaps the biggest concern at this time were the cholera epidemics of 1831–32, 1848, 1854 and 1866. Cholera is a bacterial infection caused by consuming contaminated food or water. It originated in Bengal, in India, and slowly spread across the trade routes, much like the Black Death in 1347. People knew it was coming, but hoped it would not arrive. At the time no one knew what caused cholera, or how to cure it.

> **Source G:** UK deaths from cholera
>
> 1831–32: 50,000
>
> 1848: 60,000
>
> 1854: 20,000

Typhoid

Typhoid is a bacterial infection, passed from human to human through contaminated food and water or faeces. It is caused by poor sanitation and lack of cleanliness, especially washing of hands and clothes. It had killed people since the times of the Ancient Greeks, and was especially noticeable in armies. The new industrial cities, where it was very difficult to keep clean and maintain a clean water supply, were fertile places for typhoid, and it was endemic – present virtually all the time. It was no respecter of rank. Prince Albert, husband of Queen Victoria, died in 1861 from typhoid caught from the drains at Windsor Castle.

In 1897–98 in Maidstone, Kent, an outbreak of typhoid occurred. Over 1800 people, out of a population of 34,000, caught the disease and 132 died. It was the largest single epidemic of the disease in Britain to date. There were over 200 reported cases in just the first eight days. Local medical services were overwhelmed; doctors and nurses were drafted in from across the country to deal with the disease. The cause of the disease was eventually traced to a nearby reservoir – Borming Reservoir – supplying part of the town. Once this was closed down the outbreak was brought under control.

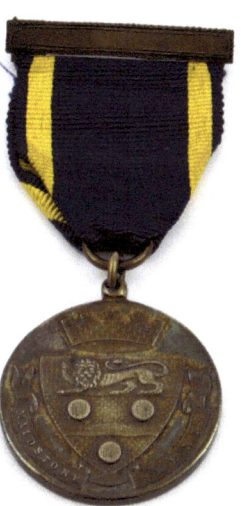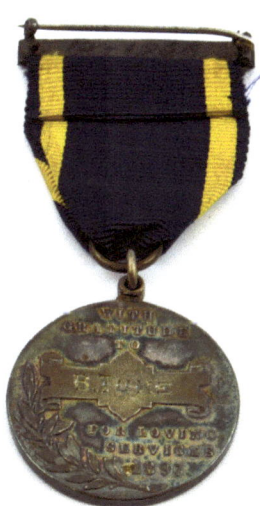

▲ **Source I:** Medal awarded to nurses who worked in Maidstone 1897–98

> **THINK**
>
> 1. Study Source H. What advice does it give to people who think they have cholera?
> 2. How does this advice compare with contemporary ideas about the spread of disease?
> 3. Look at Source I. Why do you think nurses treating typhoid in Maidstone were issued with a medal?
> 4. What does that tell us about the way people at the time thought about:
>   a) nurses and
>   b) typhoid?

▲ **Source H:** Notice issued in Limehouse in 1866 giving advice for dealing with cholera

The spread of bacterial and viral diseases in the twentieth century

In the twentieth century both bacterial and viral diseases continued to spread. The outbreak of flu after the First World War and the recent occurrence of AIDS are two examples of this. (You can find out more about how bacteria cause disease on page 40.)

Case study: a visit by 'The Spanish Lady' in 1918–19. More devastating than the Black Death?

In 1918 a flu **pandemic** spread around a war-weary world. An estimated 20–40 million people worldwide died as a result. It was a particularly devastating strain, evolved from bird flu and thought to originate in China. It is said to have infected 20 per cent of the world's population, and proved most deadly for 20–40-year olds. Initially it was thought to be a result of German biological warfare, or an effect of prolonged trench warfare and the use of mustard gas. What is clear is that mass troop movements in 1918 after the end of the First World War helped rapidly transmit the disease across the globe. Homecoming troops then spread the disease to the civilian population.

In the UK the government imposed censorship about the spread of the infection in a bid to prevent panic, but newspapers were allowed to report the seven million deaths in Spain, hence the name given to the disease: Spanish Flu, or 'The Spanish Lady'. A visit from 'the Lady' could be deadly: apparently healthy people at breakfast time could be dead by tea time. In a post-war weary and weakened population it spread rapidly, but no one knew why. Symptoms were quite general at first: headaches, sore throat and loss of appetite. Those who recovered seemed to recover quickly, so the outbreak was originally known as 'Three-Day Fever'. Hospitals could not cope. In a few months in the UK around 280,000 people died, mostly young men and women. Up to 20 per cent of those infected died. Australian troops were stationed at Sutton Veny in Wiltshire from 1915 to 1919, and there was a military hospital there. Part of the cemetery is now a Commonwealth War Graves Commission site. Many Australian victims of the flu epidemic are buried there.

> **Source K:** A children's skipping song, 1918–19
>
> *I had a little bird,*
> *it's name was Enza.*
> *I opened a window*
> *and in-flu-enza*

> **THINK**
> 1. Is it accurate to compare the 1918–19 flu pendemic with the Black Death (see page 21)?
> 2. What can we learn about the causes of illness and disease in the twentieth century from the flu pandemic?

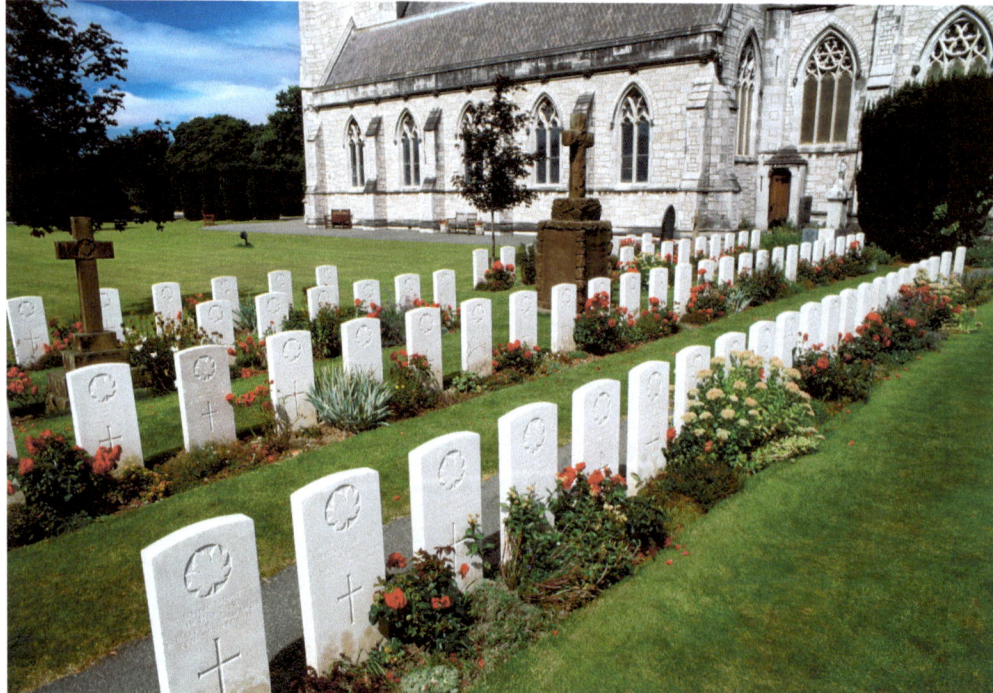

Source J: Headstones marking the graves of Canadian soldiers who fell victim to the flu epidemic, St Margarets, Clwyd

Case study: the fight against AIDS

AIDS, or Acquired Immune Deficiency Syndrome, was first identified in 1981 in the USA when doctors noticed that large numbers of gay men were dying from causes that could not easily be identified. It took until 1983 for scientists to discover that a viral infection, HIV (Human Immunodeficiency Virus), was attacking the immune system that protects the body from disease. AIDS is the most advanced stage of the HIV infection.

Since then, HIV and AIDS have spread around the world. In 2020 there were about 37.7 million people in the world with HIV; 53 per cent of these were women and girls. Deaths from AIDS are declining, and in 2020 680,000 worldwide died from the disease. In 2020 there were approximately 97,740 people living with HIV in the UK, and it is believed about 4,660 of them were unaware of their infection.

People do not die of AIDS, but often from catching very simple infections, like colds, because the weakened immune system cannot fight off infection. The most common ways to get AIDS in the UK were by having unprotected sex with someone who has the disease and by sharing hypodermic needles. It can also be transferred from mother to child during pregnancy or breast-feeding. Freddie Mercury, lead singer of the band Queen, is a high-profile person who has died of AIDS.

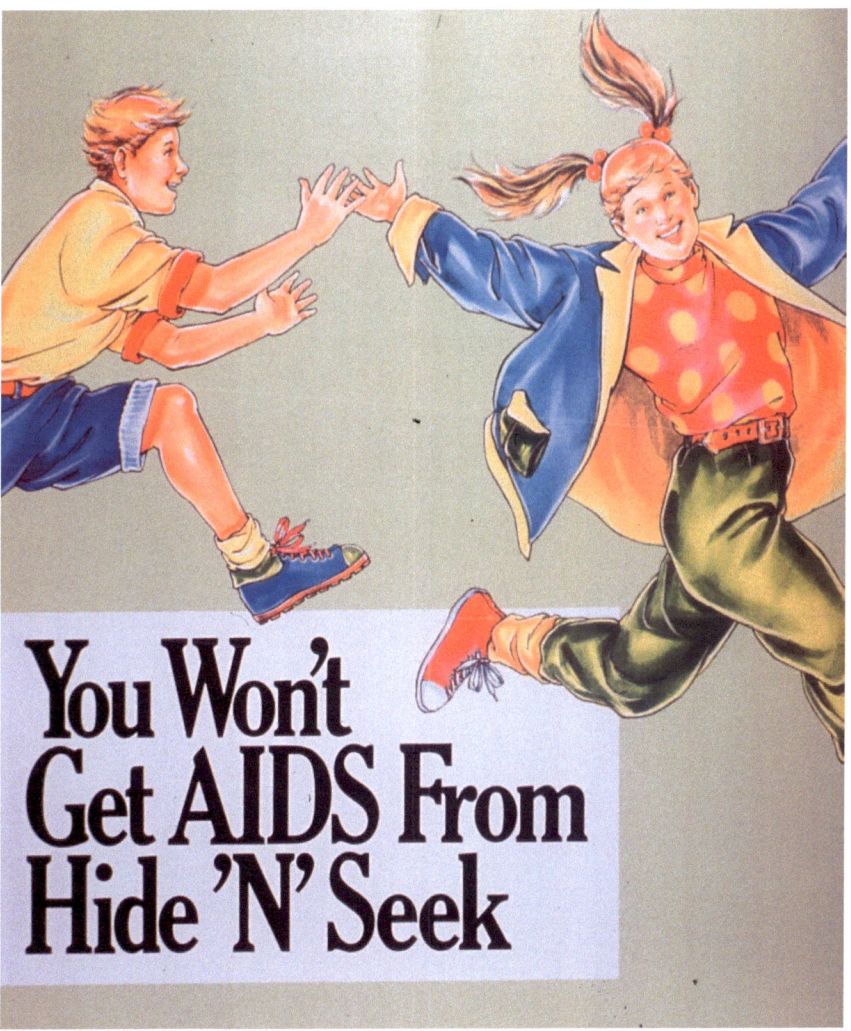

Source L: An AIDS poster from the 1980s

> **THINK**
> 1 What message is Source L trying to put across?
> 2 How is this message similar to, and different from, messages put out about the Black Death (page 21)?

In the 1980s there was still much discrimination towards gay people and much of the early reaction to AIDS reflected this. Rather than giving people practical advice on how to avoid catching HIV or what to do if you had it, health campaigns tended to be very moralistic in tone. Some people believed that sufferers had brought this disease on themselves through sexual behaviour they viewed as immoral. The health campaigns often indicated that celibacy (not having sex) was the only way to avoid contracting HIV – the poster in Source L is an example of this – and did not give advice on how to practise safe sex. It was very much viewed as a disease that only gay men or those who did drugs could get, when in fact you can get HIV through heterosexual sex.

There was a lot of misinformation about how AIDS could be transmitted – AIDS cannot be transmitted by sharing kitchen utensils, holding hands or kissing, but many believed that it could. This resulted in much discrimination and stigma around the disease and the gay community. Some of this stigma and misinformation is still around today and is a key reason why people might not get help with the condition.

Since the 1980s many people and organisations have fought to improve medical treatments for people living with HIV and AIDS and to reduce discrimination. Many of these activists were from the gay and lesbian communities, people living with HIV/AIDS themselves and people who had lost loved ones to the disease. The most prominent activist group, ACT UP, started in the USA in 1987, and had groups in the UK. They organised protests and demonstrations to help publicise and get support for those living with HIV/AIDS.

Although there is still no cure for HIV or AIDS, there are very effective drugs for controlling HIV that stop it developing into AIDS, and today many people live healthy lives with the virus. With modern drugs it is possible to reduce the level of infection in your body to such a low point that you cannot pass it on to others. In 2014 The United Nations Programme on HIV/AIDS (known as UNAIDS) set a 95-95-95 target that by 2025:

- 95 per cent of people living with HIV would know they have the virus
- 95 per cent of people living with HIV would be receiving treatment
- 95 per cent of people living with HIV would have a suppressed viral load, meaning they remained healthy and have a low risk of passing on to others.

In 2020 the UK beat these goals.

ACTIVITIES

1. Make two lists: one listing all the similarities between AIDS and the other epidemics you have studied and the other listing all the differences between AIDS and the other epidemics.
2. Compare the two lists. What conclusions can you draw?

1 Causes of illness and disease

FOCUS TASK REVISITED

1 Your focus task was to make a 'cause of illness and disease' card for every cause you came across as you worked through this chapter.
2 Take your 'cause of illness and disease' cards and sort them into categories – which are, in your opinion, the *most important* causes, and which are the least important?
3 Re-sort your 'cause of illness and disease' cards according to the time they were most important – for example, the plague might be most important in medieval times but not today.
4 What *patterns* can you discover in the causes of illness and disease?
5 Look back at the 'killer diseases of late twentieth-century Britain '(Source B, page 13), in the Big Story chapter of this book. Make 'cause of illness and disease' cards for each of those diseases too.
6 How have the causes of illness and disease changed from medieval times to today?

ACTIVITIES

Throughout history, poverty has been the main cause of illness and disease. Do you agree?

1 In pairs, prepare notes for a class debate about the causes of illness and disease. One of you can make notes agreeing that poverty was the main cause, the other can prepare notes suggesting other reasons.
2 When you have your notes, join with others who have the same view as you, and produce an agreed set of notes. Split your arguments into 'major' and 'minor', then choose two speakers to present your ideas to the rest of the class.
3 After the debate the whole class can then decide if poverty was the main cause of illness and disease.

TOPIC SUMMARY

- For much of this period many of the causes of disease were not clearly known or understood.
- Poverty and poor living conditions helped cause illness and disease throughout the period.
- Accidents remain a major cause of illness, disease and death.
- Towns were often unhealthier than the countryside.
- Epidemics continue to be a major cause of illness and disease.
- Childhood was an especially dangerous time.
- It was very difficult for people to keep clean even if they tried to.
- Warfare and famine were major causes of disease throughout the period.
- The growth of industry introduced new diseases into towns and cities.

Practice questions

1 Describe how the causes of disease have changed from c.500 to the present day. (*For guidance, see page 125.*)
2 Which of the two sources – *Anglo-Saxon Chronicle* (page 15) and the bill of mortality for London February 1664 (page 22) – is the more useful to a historian studying causes of illness and disease over time? (*For guidance, see page 123.*)
3 Outline how thinking about the causes of illness and disease have changed from the Black Death to the Plague. (*For guidance, see page 127.*)
4 Explain why the new industrial towns of the nineteenth century were so bad to live in. (*For guidance, see page 126.*)

2 Attempts to prevent illness and disease

This chapter focuses on the key question: How effective were attempts to prevent illness and disease over time?

It is very difficult to effectively prevent illness and disease when you do not really know the causes. For much of this period people could treat the symptoms of a disease, rather than the disease itself. Nevertheless, even the Ancient Greeks advocated healthy living as a means of keeping well and since then, as people increasingly identified causes of illness, as we have seen already in Chapter 1, preventative measures have become increasingly important – so much so that today as much effort is put into preventing disease as in treating it. This chapter explores attempts throughout the period of trying to prevent illness and disease.

FOCUS TASK

As you work through this chapter we would like you to build up a 'mind map' of attempts to prevent illness and disease. This will help you decide if there are any links between the different sections of this chapter, and to see if later attempts at prevention build on earlier ones. It is important that you use your 'mind map' to try to build up a 'Big Picture' of disease prevention across the whole period studied.

Early methods of prevention of disease with reference to the Black Death

The Ancient Greeks had some understanding of the prevention of disease. Hippocrates was born in Kos, in Greece, in 460BC. He is regarded by many as the father of modern medicine and was perhaps the first physician to regard and treat the body as a whole, rather than as individual parts. Hippocrates based his thinking and writing around the theory of the **four humours**. In order to prevent illness and disease all you had to do was to keep the four humours of blood, phlegm, yellow bile and black bile in balance. Hippocrates also believed diet, exercise and rest had a huge part to play in prevention of disease. The Arabs believed in the importance of cleanliness and fresh air and the Romans built huge aqueducts to bring fresh water to their towns, with most Roman villas having a bath and toilet with running water. However, much of this was lost when the Romans left Britain around AD410. Most medieval physicians continued to be trained in, and believed in, the theory of the four humours. (We will be exploring the theory of the four humours in more detail in Chapter 4.)

The role of the church

The church was very influential in medieval times, and it argued that physical illness was a manifestation of spiritual illness. In other words, people became ill because they were either living in an unchristian way or they were not praying hard enough. To stop the Black Death the church ordered people to take part in processions through towns and villages to the local church, and pray for forgiveness. Some people took this further: they made life-size candles and burned those in church, asking to be spared. Others took to walking around the streets whipping themselves in order to purify themselves in God's eyes, and thus hope to be spared from the Black Death.

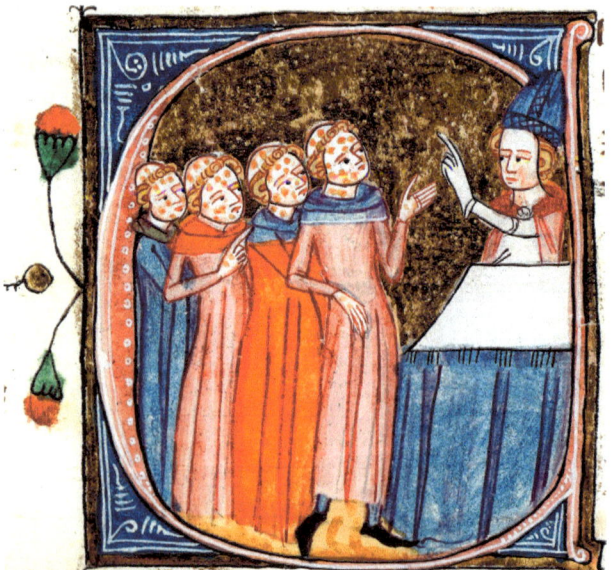

▲ **Source A:** Monks with the plague being blessed by a priest from a fourteenth-century manuscript

Other attempts to prevent catching the Black Death

Many other suggestions were made if you wanted to avoid the Black Death. Some argued you should not eat too much, or you should not bathe. Having a bath opened the pores of the skin and allowed disease into the body. Some said washing would keep you clean and keep the Black Death away! Others suggested avoiding sex, as having sex weakened the body's defences against illness, or drinking vinegar and/or wine; drinking urine once a day; bathing in urine three times a day; bleeding to let out the evil spirits that might cause disease; killing all the cats and dogs as they spread disease; even carrying a posy of sweet-smelling herbs with you as this would stop the bad smell that some thought caused the disease. Putting coins in vinegar when paying for your shopping was also thought to prevent passing on the disease.

Some people came closer to effective prevention, without really knowing why. King Edward III ordered the streets of London cleaned of all the filth, arguing that the smell spread the Black Death. Other more practical advice was to avoid coming into contact with people who had the disease. House doors of those with the Black Death were often boarded up and a big red cross painted on them, warning people to keep away. Many people attempted to avoid the Black Death by fleeing – but unwittingly all this did was to help spread the Black Death even further.

As you can see from the proposed preventative measures, and as you already learned in Chapter 1, no-one really knew what to do to stop the Black Death spreading, or to keep people safe from it.

> **THINK**
>
> 1. Which of the preventative measures suggested do you think might have helped people avoid the Black Death? Why?
> 2. What do all these suggestions tell us about medieval attempts to prevent illness and disease?
> 3. Look at Source A. How can you tell these monks have the Black Death? Why is the priest blessing them?
> 4. Look at Source B. It is from a fourteenth-century prayer book and was painted in 1376. What do images like this tell us about attempts to prevent catching the Black Death?
> 5. What do Sources A and B tell us about medieval attitudes to the prevention of illness and disease?

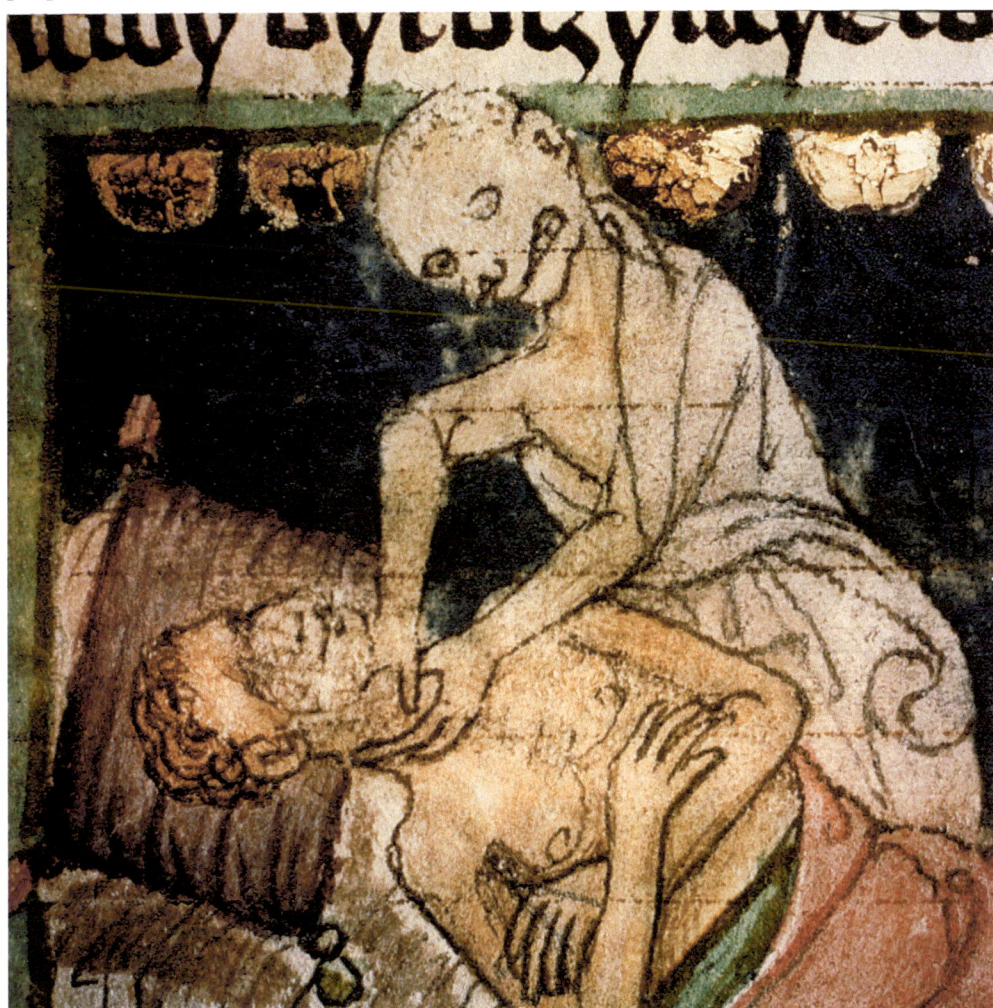

▲ **Source B:** Death strangling a victim of the Black Death, painted by Werner Forman in 1376

Alchemy, soothsayers and medieval doctors

> **THINK**
> 1. To what extent did alchemy help the prevention of illnesses and disease?
> 2. Look at Source C. How has the artist chosen to portray the alchemist?
> 3. How useful is Source C to understanding of the part played by alchemy in preventing disease?

Alchemy

There was often very little difference between scientists and alchemists in medieval and early modern times. Some of the most eminent scientists – Roger Bacon in the thirteenth century, Isaac Newton in the seventeenth century, for example – delved into alchemy. Most of their experiments were attempts to turn 'base' metals such as lead into gold, but many scientific discoveries were made by these experiments, although no one managed to create gold from another substance. These scientific discoveries became important later, and helped others, such as William Harvey, in their work (see page 58).

Alchemists by their nature tended to be secretive about their experiments, and so all kinds of stories grew about them, about what they were doing, and what they had achieved. Many were searching for the 'Elixir of Life', which was supposed to keep you young forever. One alchemist claimed to be 1000 years old but when pushed for evidence could give no proof. Obviously if you could discover this Elixir of Life you could make a fortune and ensure everyone could be free from illness and old age. This new medicine, or 'quintessence' as it was known, often made by repeatedly distilling vinegar, was meant to remove all impurities from the body. Sometimes strong medicines containing poisons, such antimony or mercury, would be used to make a patient violently sick, thus being seen to prevent disease.

Gullible people were prepared to advance large sums of money to alchemists in exchange for turning lead into gold or for providing longer life. John Dee (1527–1608/9) was an adviser to Queen Elizabeth I and a famous mathematician. He was also a famous astronomer. From 1580 onwards he spent much of his time investigating the world of magic, trying to discover how to communicate with angels, in order to find out more about the Creation of the Earth by God. He did not see a distinction between his mathematical investigations and his study of magic and demons or his search for the secret of long life. Gerard of York, Archbishop of York until his death in 1108, was reported to be a student of the 'dark arts', magic and medicine although this may have been more a result of his attempts to reform the church against the wishes of his clergy than his own interests.

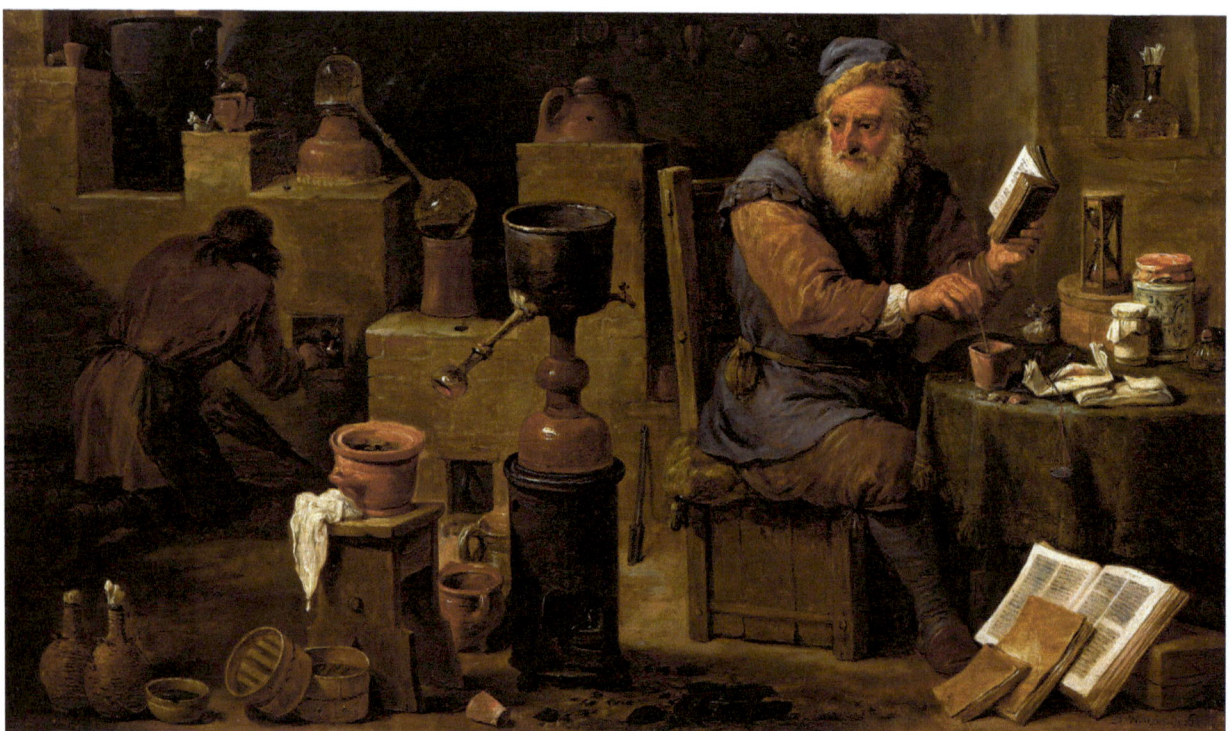

▲ **Source C:** *The Alchemist*, by David Teniers the Younger, seventeenth century

Soothsayers

There were very few qualified doctors in medieval England. Most people would depend on the local 'wise woman'. These would build up knowledge of sickness and disease over several generations, and each would have their own favourite methods. Some of them might even work! Soothsayers were also supposed to have powers of prophesy – to be able to see the future, and were often consulted by local people for a variety of purposes. They would collect plants and herbs, special stones, anything that might help, and carry this about with them in a willow basket. They would, for a price, put together special charms to be worn as protection against evil. Remember, the church strongly argued that most illness and disease was caused by evil, or by not living a Christian enough life.

Case study: can we believe most of what was written about Mother Shipton?

Mother Shipton became famous as a fifteenth-century soothsayer. She was born in a cave near Knaresborough, in Yorkshire, around the year 1488 and died around 1561. You can still visit the cave today. It is one of Yorkshire's top tourist attractions. Next to the cave is a petrifying well – the only one in England – where the water has a high mineral content. Drinking it, or bathing in it, was said to keep you fit and healthy. From the sixteenth century people have visited the well for that purpose.

Mother Shipton is said to have been extremely ugly, but she gained quite a reputation for prophesying events. Local people came to her, then people from across the whole of Yorkshire and, eventually, from the whole of England. Her prophesies were first published in 1641, where this illustration of her is thought to have come from. Each subsequent edition of her prophesies included more and more predictions for the future, including that the world would end in 1881, or 1891, or 1981, depending on which version you believed!

She is perhaps a famous – or should that be infamous – example of many local soothsayers that we know nothing about, but who played an important part in helping medieval people avoid illness and disease.

Medieval doctors

As we have seen already, doctors were few and far between in medieval England. There were monks before Henry VIII abolished the monasteries in 1536 who would provide simple medical care; there were apothecaries who made up their own herbal remedies; there were barber-surgeons who might pull out a bad tooth or set a broken arm (see page 44); and there were physicians, probably trained at one of the new universities in Italy or Paris. Unfortunately, very few of them knew much about prevention of disease, because so little was known about causes of disease.

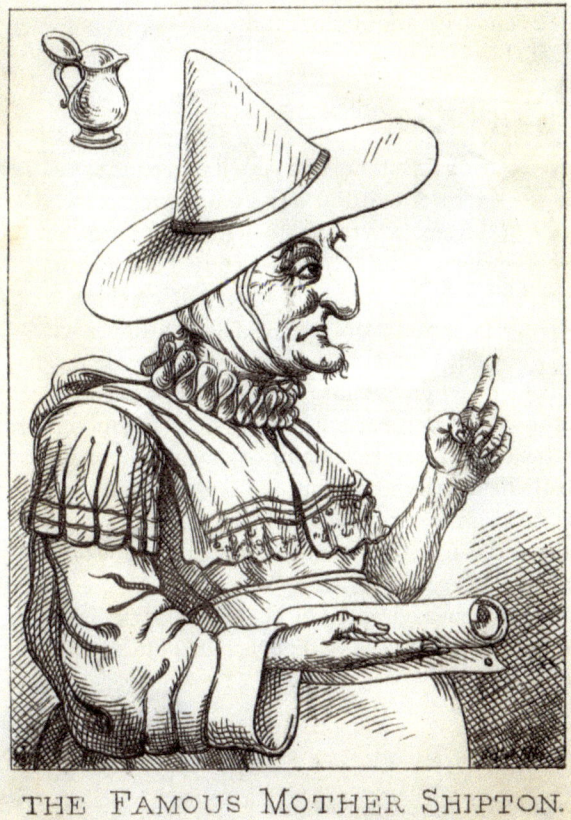

▲ **Source D:** A seventeenth-century engraving said to be of Mother Shipton

> ### THINK
> 1. How accurate a depiction of Mother Shipton do you think this is?
> 2. How useful is Source D in finding out about Mother Shipton?
> 3. Does Source D prove that Mother Shipton existed? Explain your decision.
> 4. In what way does Source D help us understand how Mother Shipton, and soothsayers, helped prevent disease?
> 5. Which, in your opinion, were the most successful methods of preventing disease in medieval times?
> 6. How effective were medieval attempts to prevent disease?

The application of science to the prevention of disease in the late eighteenth and early nineteenth centuries

'Prevention is better than cure!'

During the eighteenth century this saying began to be heard more and more, as people rediscovered the Classical World, and the Ancient Greek's belief in fresh air, exercise and diet. John Bellers produced a book in 1714, his *Essay towards the Improvement of Physick* in which he argued that 100,000 people died each year 'for want of timely advice and suitable medicine'. It was a time of fads. Vegetarianism became fashionable, as did teetotalism. Both would keep you healthy and prevent disease. Regular bloodletting would prevent an imbalance of the four humours building up. Fresh air and exercise were all the rage – at least for those with the time and money to indulge it.

The cold water treatment

'Taking the cure' at a spa became part of the season. It was widely believed that the waters of places such as Buxton and Bath were beneficial to health and were preventative measures as well as cures. Visiting the seaside, places such as Bognor Regis and Brighton, and swimming in the ocean was recommended to keep you healthy. It became fashionable to have your own 'plunge pool' of cold fresh water in the garden – as near to a source of fresh water as possible – and this was the perfect end to a brisk walk around the estate. Later in the period, the water would be piped inside the house and cold water bathing indoors became the trend. Eating 'cooling' foods was regarded as an essential part of the therapy. Drinking at least a litre of cold water every morning was supposed to clear out the impurities from the bowels that caused illness and disease. Many wealthier people in the eighteenth and nineteenth centuries adopted such measures in a bid to remain healthy.

Child-bed fever

As we have seen, childbirth was a very dangerous time for women. Alexander Gordon was a naval surgeon who worked in London for several years before returning to his native Aberdeen. While there he studied an outbreak of child-bed fever and worked out what caused these deaths. He noticed that women in outlying villages who were treated by the village wise woman or midwife rarely caught the fever, whereas those treated by doctors or midwives moving from patient to patient were much more likely to die. He realised that he himself was responsible for some of the deaths. His proposed cure was simple: medical practitioners ought to wash their clothes frequently, and wash their hands in chlorinated water to try to limit the spread of disease. When he published his results in 1795 he was derided by the whole of the medical profession and it was many years before his ideas were implemented.

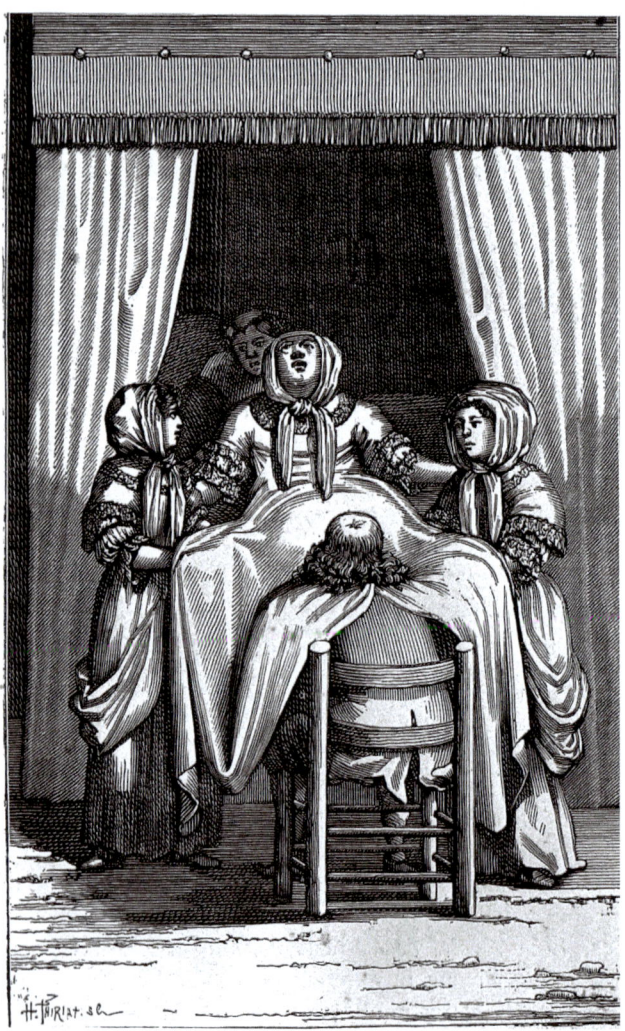

▲ **Source E:** An engraving depicting childbirth in the eighteenth century

> **THINK**
> 1. How effective, in your opinion, are these 'fads' and 'cures' at preventing disease?
> 2. Study Source E. Can you identify any factors likely to cause either harm or death to the mother or newborn child? Do you think the midwife is familiar with the ideas of Alexander Gordon? How can you tell?

The rise of the scientific method

A series of inventions helped people keep healthy. The microscope (for seeing infections), the stethoscope (for listening to a patient's breathing) and the kymograph (for measuring blood pressure) all became part of a doctor's armoury in the early nineteenth century, allowing better investigation of health. Many scientific papers were published. James Lind, for example, identified the cause of scurvy in 1753. He insisted that sailors be given doses of lime juice and/or fresh fruit every day to keep them healthy (hence English sailors' nickname as 'Limeys'). During the eighteenth century many texts were written as a result of extensive scientific investigation of illnesses. These papers were published in order to bring about better treatment and prevention.

John Snow and cholera

Perhaps the greatest example of the application of science to disease prevention in the nineteenth century was the work of John Snow in London in 1854, during the cholera epidemic. Cholera, as we saw in Chapter 1 (page 25) was one of the killer diseases of the nineteenth century. John Snow, a London physician, carefully plotted on a street plan each and every cholera case in the area around his surgery (Figure 2.1). Within a few weeks over 500 deaths occurred in the neighbourhood of Broad Street.

He noticed that in a nearby area, where there was a brewery, the brewery workers didn't catch cholera, because they drank beer rather than water. He used statistics to illustrate the link between the quality of the water from different sources and cholera deaths. He thus showed that the Southwark and Vauxhall Waterworks Company was taking water from sewage-polluted sections of the Thames and delivering the water to homes with an increased incidence of cholera. He came to the conclusion – without being able to decisively prove why – that the source of the local infection was one particular water pump in Broad Street. When he took the handle off the pump – forcing residents to obtain their water elsewhere – the disease declined.

▲ **Source F:** Poster issued in 1854 telling people how to prevent being infected by cholera

> **THINK**
> 1. According to Source F, how do you avoid getting cholera?
> 2. Do what extent does this agree with the ideas of John Snow?
> 3. What does Source F tell us about ideas of preventing disease in the nineteenth century?
> 4. Are they any different to earlier times?
> 5. What impact do you think the scientific method had on prevention of illness and disease in the eighteenth and nineteenth centuries?

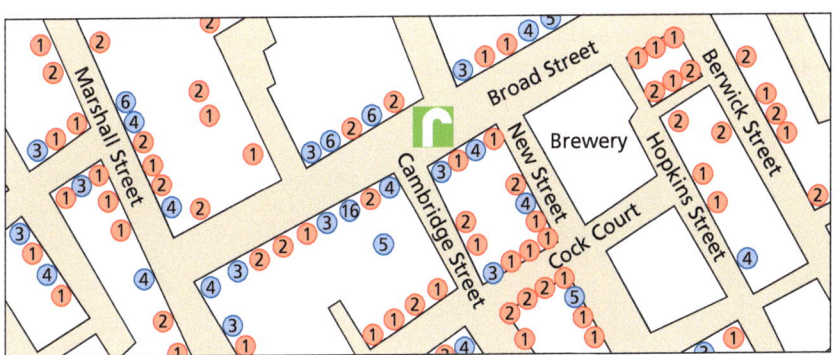

◀ Figure 2.1: A copy of part of Snow's map detailing deaths in the Broad Street area

The work of Edward Jenner and vaccination

The story of Dr Jenner is inspirational – an inspired guess, based on experiment and scientific method, produced a vaccine that protected people from one of the most deadly infectious diseased of the period. And yet Jenner was ridiculed as a country doctor and vaccination questioned as an effective method of controlling smallpox – an argument still reflected today in the debate about the utility of vaccination in preventing disease.

Smallpox

Smallpox is an acute contagious disease caused by the variola virus. It was one of the world's most devastating diseases. It was declared eradicated in 1980 following a global vaccination campaign led by the World Health Organization. But in earlier times it was an absolute killer. Between 30 and 60 per cent of those who caught smallpox died. Survivors carried the legacies of smallpox for life. Some were left blind; virtually all were disfigured by scars. Smallpox had long been endemic in Britain, and had been a feared killer since the seventeenth century. Major epidemics had killed at least 35,000 in 1796, and 42,000 between 1837 and 1840. The disease was no respecter of rank – Queen Mary died of smallpox in 1694. People thought it was caused by miasma, or 'bad air'.

Vaccination is not new – it dates from the eighteenth century. And inoculation has been used long before that, being widely used in the Far East for many centuries. Lady Mary Montagu came across it in Istanbul and introduced it to England in 1721. Her husband had been Ambassador to the Ottoman Empire and she had seen it used there. She had personally survived a smallpox outbreak that killed her brother and left her scarred. Basically, a mild form of smallpox was introduced into a scratch made between finger and thumb. The person being inoculated then developed a mild form of the disease, but became immune to the stronger version of smallpox. When smallpox broke out in England Lady Montagu had her children inoculated. And it worked.

A country doctor changes everything …

Edward Jenner, a country doctor in Gloucestershire who had studied in London, heard the local gossips say that milkmaids who caught cowpox never seemed to catch smallpox. He reasoned that having cowpox must give them immunity from smallpox, but how could he prove it? He experimented on local people. He chose a nine-year-old boy, James Phipps, who had had neither cowpox nor smallpox. He injected him with pus from the sores of a milkmaid with cowpox. James developed cowpox. Later, when he had recovered, Jenner gave him a dose of smallpox. James was immune. Jenner had proved that an injection of cowpox stopped people catching smallpox. He knew it worked, but didn't know how! He submitted a paper to the Royal Society in 1797 but was told he needed more proof. So he carried out more experiments, including on his own 11-month-old son, all the time keeping detailed notes and records.

Finally, in 1798, Jenner published *An Inquiry into the Causes and Effects of the Variolæ Vaccinæ, or Cow-Pox*. He continued to work on vaccination and in 1802 was awarded £10,000 by the government for his work, and a further £20,000 in 1807 after the Royal College of Physicians confirmed how effective vaccination was.

What impact did vaccination have on smallpox?

Reaction to Jenner and his work was mixed. Those who charged up to £20 a time to inoculate patients saw that their livelihoods were threatened, and poured scorn on the whole idea of change. Many people felt it was wrong to inject cowpox into humans. Some argued that smallpox was God's punishment for living a sinful life and so we should not interfere, or limit the spread of the disease. Others thought it should be up to parents to decide whether their children should be treated or not. Yet others – some actually in favour of vaccination, others opposed to it – felt strongly it was not the government's job to interfere in such things. In 1840, partly as a result of the dreadful epidemic of 1837–40, vaccination was made free to all infants, and in 1852 it was made compulsory, but not strictly enforced. It seems strange that a laissez-faire government, which was reluctant to interfere in most aspects of life, would make vaccination compulsory. This, surely, tells us a lot about the fear of smallpox as a killer disease. There was an anti-vaccine league set up in England in 1866, to oppose the idea of compulsory vaccination (see Source H on page 38). It was not until 1871 that the government became much stricter – parents could be fined for not having their children vaccinated. Once the death rate fell dramatically the government in 1887 introduced the right for parents to refuse vaccination.

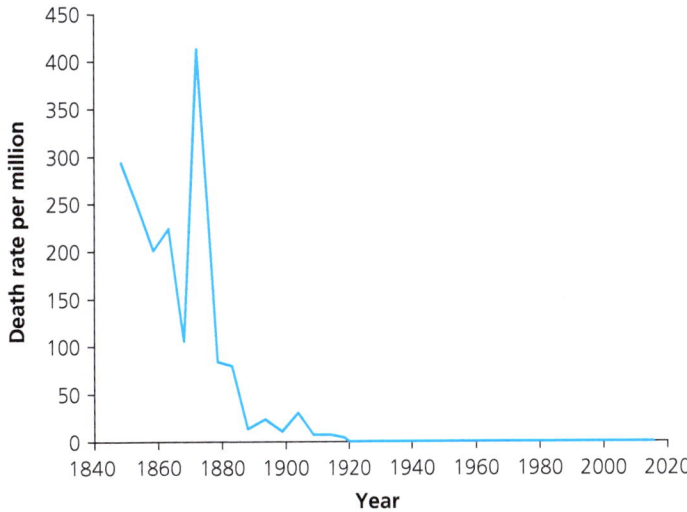

▲ Figure 2.2: Graph showing deaths from smallpox, 1848–1920

THINK

1. Why was smallpox so deadly?
2. What is the difference between inoculation and vaccination?
3. Is Source G pro-Jenner or anti-Jenner? How can you tell?
4. What part did chance, government, science and technology or the role of the individual play in the discovery of a cure for smallpox?
5. How does the work of Jenner help us understand the world of medicine in early modern Britain?
6. Is vaccination a 'success story'?
7. Why do you think the government made vaccination compulsory?

▼ Source G: Edward Jenner vaccinating patients against smallpox

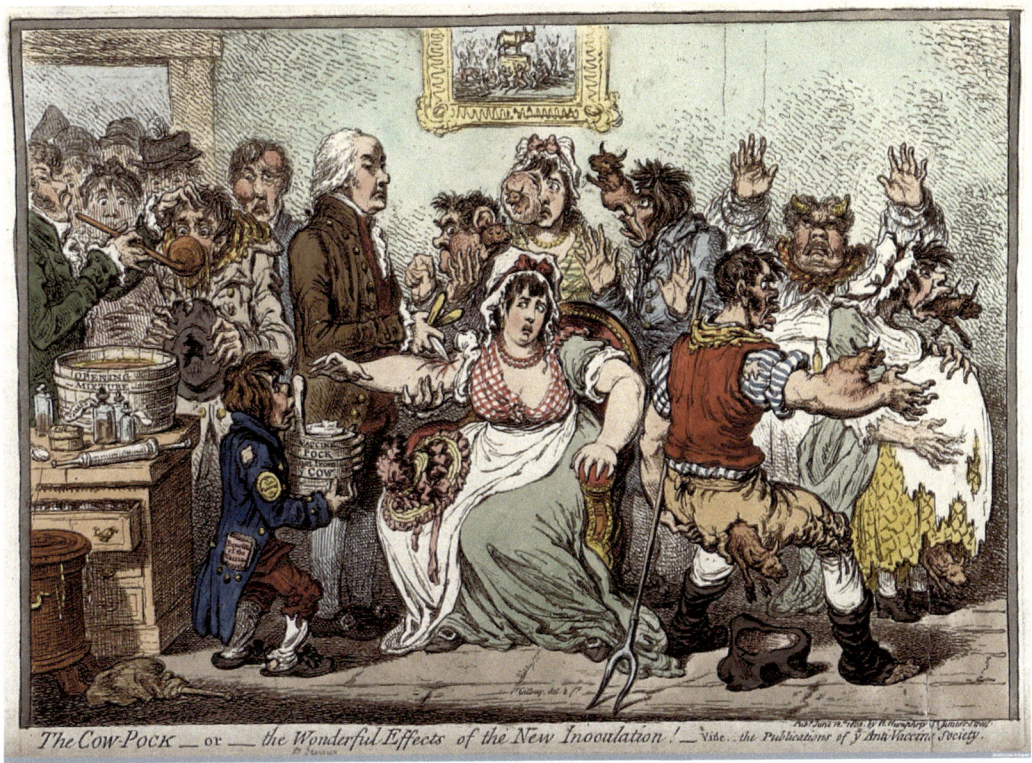

The influence and spread of inoculation since 1700

In the twentieth century, what were once endemic diseases and childhood killers, such as polio, measles, diphtheria and whooping cough, had almost been eliminated through vaccination programmes. The World Health Organization has led the campaign to eliminate these diseases throughout the world. The last known case of smallpox was in Somalia in 1977 – quite a success story and all stemming from on the work of Edward Jenner in a small country town in Gloucestershire.

In England more and more vaccines have been introduced since the Second World War. Polio vaccine was introduced in 1955, measles in 1963, MMR (measles, mumps and rubella) in 1988 and Hepatitis B in 1994. If we are travelling abroad it is now common to receive anti-malaria and anti-yellow fever vaccinations. There are vaccinations for babies, for children, for young adults and for pregnant women. All these have had a profound impact on what were once killer diseases. The infant mortality rate has fallen dramatically – in 1800 it averaged over 150 per thousand, by 1900 this had risen to around 170 per thousand, whereas today it is between 4 and 5 deaths per thousand live births (see Figure 2.3). Much, but not all, of this fall is down to the effects of immunisation.

Yet the very success of immunisation has led to debate about whether or not government has the right to impose vaccinations on us.

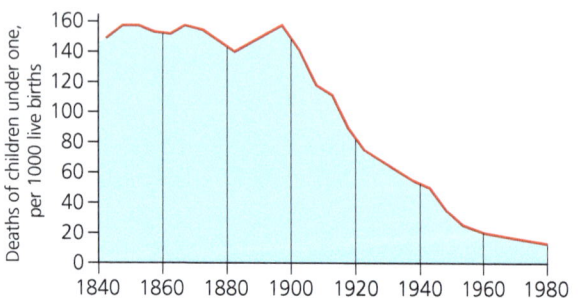

▲ Figure 2.3: The rate of infant mortaility (the death rate of children under one years old), 1840–1980

MEN AND WOMEN OF THE TOWER HAMLETS,
And all who value Parental Liberty!
MR. THOMAS ERNEST WISE
Of 31 Clayhill Road, Bow
HAS BEEN IMPRISONED
for 10 days at the behest of the
VILE, FILTHY, VACCINATION LAW.
HE WILL BE
LIBERATED ON SATURDAY, SEPT. 27th.
Mr. WISE has been fighting a battle for freedom on behalf of Thousands of parents.

It is intended to give Mr. WISE a warm welcome on his return home, and to show him that We honour
Our First Vaccination Martyr.

▲ Source H: A poster from the 1870s

> **THINK**
> 1 What does Figure 2.3 tell us about the following:
>   ☐ infant mortality
>   ☐ inoculation
>   ☐ health
>   ☐ prevention of disease.
> 2 Look at Source H.
>   ☐ What did some Victorians think about vaccination?
>   ☐ Why were they opposed to vaccination law?
> 3 Look at Source I (on page 39).
>   ☐ Why is this author in favour of vaccination?
>   ☐ How similar and how different are the ideas used in each of these sources?

The MMR debate

In 1998 Dr Wakefield published a paper in the *Lancet*, a medical journal in Britain, suggesting there was a clear link between the MMR routinely given to all young children and autism. It claimed that evidence from his small study showed that being vaccinated with the MMR vaccine led, in some cases, to the development of autism. Even though they were only preliminary results, unverified by any other researcher, the press made a huge story out of it, and the proportion of parents having their children vaccinated plummeted. To be successful 95 per cent of the target population must be vaccinated, otherwise there is a chance of someone with the disease passing it on to others, and an epidemic can break out.

Since then a fierce debate about vaccination has raged, both here in the UK and around the world.

> **Source I:** Extract from the *Guardian*, 3 February 2015
>
> *To the anti-vaxxers: please don't give measles to my tiny, helpless future baby.*
>
> *Herd immunity isn't about my individual hypothetical baby, or yours – it's about public health, investing in a collective. It's a testament to the idea that we can care about human life independent of self-interest. That empathy extends beyond our own children ...*

In effect, the argument is about choice – do I have the choice, as a parent, not to have my baby vaccinated? There is plenty of evidence that for some, about one per cent of children, vaccines produce a reaction. These are not usually very serious – the UK Vaccine Payment Fund, set up to pay compensation to those badly affected by vaccination, has paid out 20 times in the last ten years – but reactions can be serious. But if you put that against the decline, and in some cases, disappearance, of highly infectious diseases then most people think vaccination a good thing. Except, of course, if you think vaccination is wrong, or that vaccines are poison, or that they are used by big business to generate vast profits from unnecessary medicines. What is noticeable is that the UK had its first major outbreak of measles in 2012–13. Vaccination rates in the UK remain around 93 per cent – not enough to ensure immunity.

Dr Wakefield's study has since been repudiated by the medical world, and shown to be bad science. But the uncertainty it has caused led to many people distrusting all vaccines and the re-emergence of some diseases the World Health Organization had declared eliminated.

THINK
1. What was Dr Wakefield arguing?
2. How carefully researched was his report?
3. What impact did his study have?
4. Do you think that the debate on inoculation is because the policy has been so successful that we no longer remember how deadly these diseases are?

The discovery of antibodies and developments in the field of bacteriology

As we have seen, both Edward Jenner and John Snow made massive strides in preventing disease without really being able to prove scientifically why their methods worked. All this changed with the work of Louis Pasteur and Robert Koch in the late nineteenth century.

Louis Pasteur, Robert Koch and germ theory

Louis Pasteur was a French scientist working in Paris. He discovered germ theory, and this changed medicine for ever. He proved that tiny organisms called bacteria caused many diseases and so to prevent disease all you had to do was kill the bacteria. Robert Koch, a German, took this work a step further as he began to identify the specific bacteria that caused specific diseases, thus making the science of bacteriology possible. Koch also realised that antibodies – a natural defence mechanism of the body against germs – could help to destroy bacteria and build up an immunity against the disease, thus keeping the body free from illness and disease. The discovery that each antibody worked specifically on only one bacteria was crucial to an understanding of how the body fought off disease. If you could introduce a weakened form of the disease into the body, as Jenner did with cowpox, then, when the deadly version of the disease attacked, the body would be able to resist. You can find out more about the work of Pasteur, Koch and his student Ehrlich in Chapter 4 (page 59).

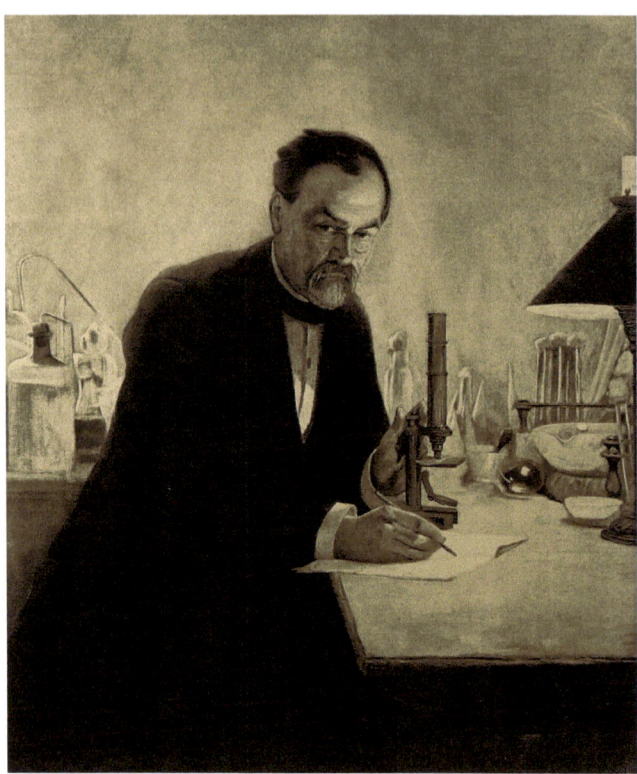

▲ Source J: Louis Pasteur

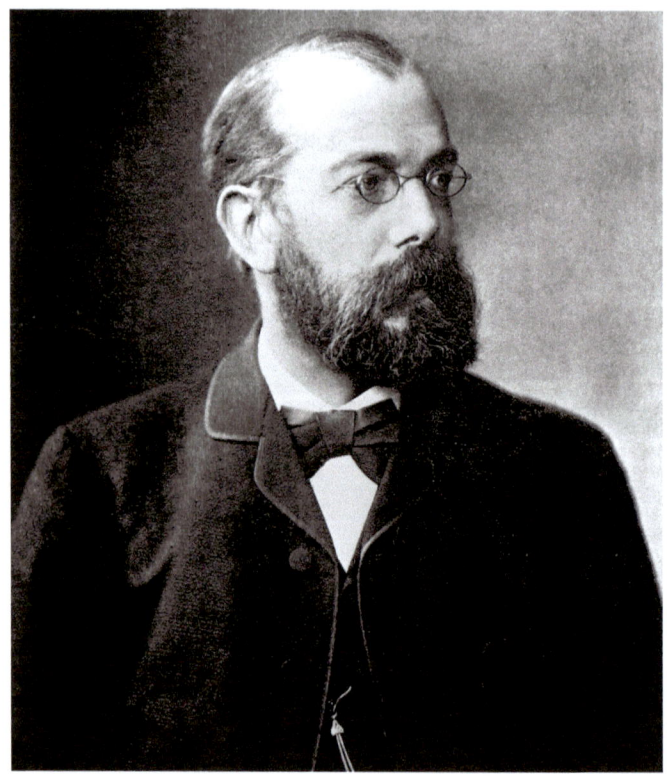

▲ Source K: Robert Koch

> **THINK**
> 1 How important is science in improving disease prevention?
> 2 Who played the bigger part in advancing preventative medicine, Pasteur or Koch?

FOCUS TASK REVISITED

1 As you worked through this chapter you will have built up a 'mind map' of attempts to prevent illness and disease. This should now help you decide if there are any links between the different sections of this chapter, and see if later attempts at prevention build on earlier ones. It is important that you use your 'mind map' to try to build up a 'Big Picture' of disease prevention across the whole period studied.
2 Use your mind map to work out *how effective* preventive efforts have been. When were they most effective? Least effective?
3 Finally, try to find links between your ideas about prevention of illness and disease and the 'causes of disease' cards you made for Chapter 1. Are there any obvious links you can make, or are they really two separate topics?

ACTIVITIES

1 Draw an annotated timeline, from AD500 to today, across the middle of a page, showing the attempts to prevent illness you have investigated in this chapter.
2 Place any attempts to prevent illness and disease that you think were successful *above* your timeline; and attempts to prevent illness and disease that you think were particularly unsuccessful *below* your timeline.
3 When, in your opinion, were attempts to prevent disease and illness *most* successful? Why?

TOPIC SUMMARY

- In the medieval period there were lots of suggestions on how to prevent illness and disease, but no-one really knew how to do so.
- Living a decent Christian life was thought to be very important, as important as exercise and diet.
- As science developed, so scientific method came closer to identifying the best ways to prevent disease.
- Jenner and Snow came up with effective preventative measures, but were unsure why they worked.
- Pasteur and Koch made the real scientific breakthrough – all work since then has been based on their discoveries.
- Alchemists spent many hours searching for the key to eternal life, without finding it.
- King Edward III ordered the streets of London cleaned, thus making a link between dirt and disease.
- People could produce and sell anything, without restriction, claiming to be able to prevent disease.
- Some people still argue today about the effectiveness of vaccination.

Practice questions

1 Describe the way medieval practitioners tried to prevent illness and disease. *(For guidance, see page 125.)*
2 Which of Source F, the cholera poster on page 35, and Source C, the painting of an alchemist by David Teniers on page 32, is the more reliable to a historian investigating prevention of illness and disease? *(For guidance, see page 123.)*
3 Explain why developments in vaccination were important in the prevention of illness and disease in the nineteenth and twentieth centuries. *(For guidance, see page 126.)*
4 Outline how attempts to prevent illness and disease have changed from c.500 to the present day. *(For guidance, see page 127.)*

3 Attempts to treat and cure illness and disease

This chapter focuses on the key question: How have attempts to treat illness and disease changed over time?

Throughout history, people have fallen ill, and doctors of various types and specialisms have attempted to cure them, perhaps not always successfully. Increasingly a scientific approach, based on observation, experimentation and measuring has led to new discoveries, medicines and techniques that have improved the chances of a successful cure, although some people today seem to prefer natural or alternative cures. This chapter looks at these changing attempts to treat and cure illness.

FOCUS TASK

As you work through this chapter, carefully make a note of each cure for an illness you come across and add it to your copy of the table below. The first one has been done for you. That way you will build up a detailed list of the different ways of treating illness mentioned. You will need the final two columns when you revisit the focus task at the end of this chapter.

Illness or disease	Cure		
Headache	Drink camomile tea and lie down		

Traditional treatments and remedies common in the medieval era

Herbal medicines

Herbs were widely used as remedies for a variety of ailments in the medieval period. Herbal medicines often contained ingredients such as honey and a mixture of other plants that we now know do help cure infections. Sometimes herbal treatments were written down in books called 'herbals' with pictures of the ingredients and explanations of the exact quantities of each ingredient and how to mix the potion. They included prayers to say while collecting the herbs to increase the effectiveness of the remedy. There were also guides as to when to pick the herbs – some recipes would only work if the ingredients were picked on the night of a full moon, or when the moon was waning, or similar. If picked at the wrong time this would mean the herbal remedy would not work. Herbal remedies were also often closely guarded family secrets, handed down through generations from mother to daughter.

> **Source A:** A cure for headache, from an early fourteenth-century book from Venice
>
> Drink warm camomile tea and then lie down on rosemary and lavender-scented pillows for fifteen minutes.

> **Source B:** Advice from Rycharde Banckes, a late medieval herbalist
>
> Gather leaves of rosemary and boyle them in fayre water and drinke that water for it is much worthe against all manner of evils in the body.

> **Source C:** Instructions to prepare an ointment, from *The Knight With the Lion* by Helen Lynch, based on medieval French stories of King Arthur
>
> Take equal amounts of radish, bishopwort, garlic, wormwood, helenium, cropleek and hollowleek. Pound them up, and boil them in butter with celandine and red nettle. Keep the mixture in a brass pot until it is a dark red colour. Strain it through a cloth and smear on the forehead or aching joints.

> **Source D:** Bald's *Leechbook*, an Anglo-Saxon (nine or tenth century) cure for a stye in the eye
>
> Take equal amounts of onion/leek and garlic, and pound them well together. Take equal amounts of wine and bull's gall and mix them with the onion and garlic. Put the mixture in a brass bowl and let it stand for nine nights, then strain it through a cloth. Then, about night-time, apply it to the eye with a feather.

> **Source E:** A Welsh thirteenth-century cure for toothache
>
> Take a candle of sheep' suet, some eringo (sea holly [Eryngium maritimum]) seed being mixed therewith, and burn it as near the tooth as possible, some cold water being held under the candle. The worms (destroying the tooth) will drop into the water, in order to escape from the heat of the candle.

3 Attempts to treat and cure illness and disease

Other common medieval remedies

Bleeding
The most favoured way to fight illness, and restore the balance of the four humours, was by bleeding. This was done either by 'cupping' (see Source F) or by using leeches (see page 44). Monastery records show some monks were bled up to eight times a year. Illness was said to be caused by the body creating too much blood so it was obvious that bleeding patients would restore their vitality. Purging was also used to rid the body of excess liquid and impurities.

Urine in diagnosis and prescription
Doctors had one other indispensible tool for diagnosing sickness and putting it right. Urine was a vital diagnostic tool. The physician would look carefully at the colour and compare it to a chart (see Source G). He might smell it and, in some circumstances, taste it to help him decide what was wrong with the patient. The remedy prescribed would then depend on the diagnosis. Again, many patients today still have to submit a urine sample as part of the process of deciding what is wrong with them.

Zodiac chart
Finally, no self-respecting physician would visit a patient without his most important tool of all – a zodiac chart (see Source H). Charts like this would tell a physician which parts of the body were linked to which astrological sign, and thus dictate what he might do to cure a patient – some things might work for an Aries, for example, but not for a Pisces. It might also tell him when was the best time to carry out his treatment, and even when to pick the herbs used in medicines – herbs picked at the wrong time of the moon's cycle, for example, might do more harm than good. It was a complicated business for physicians to decide what was causing an illness and how it might best be treated.

Other treatments
And of course there were still plenty of 'quacks' or unlicensed traders who roamed around the country, visiting out-of-the-way places and appearing at markets and fairs, offering all kinds of treatment and cures – some better than others.

> **THINK**
> 1. Look at Sources A–E. Do you think any of these cures were effective? Rank them in order of how well you think they work. Explain the order you have chosen.
> 2. Would they do any harm?
> 3. How would medieval people learn about such cures?

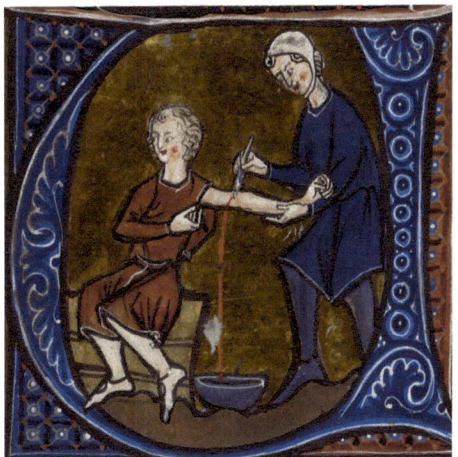

▲ **Source F:** Bloodletting, from an illuminated medieval manuscript

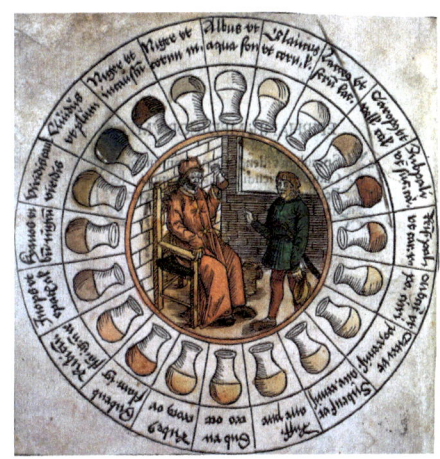

▲ **Source G:** A urine chart used by physicians in the medieval period

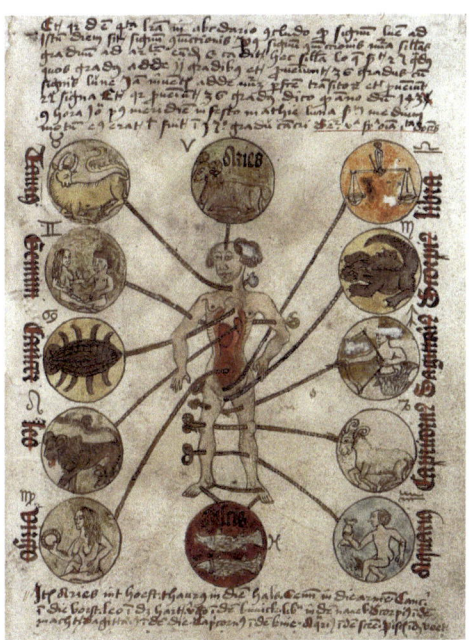

▲ **Source H:** A zodiac chart from the fifteenth century

Barber-surgeons and the use of leeches

In the medieval period surgeons were mostly barber-surgeons, with little training or medical knowledge, save that gained by an apprenticeship and experience. You would find barber-surgeons in most towns. They would pull teeth, mend broken limbs, carry out bloodletting as well as cut your hair (see Source I). They would also carry out simple surgery. Sometimes they might combine their trade with that of apothecary, producing herbal medicines of various degrees of effectiveness. They might be the only medical professional available to many people, certainly to those who could not afford a physician.

The use of leeches

Leeches have been used in medicine for over 2500 years. They slowly suck blood, in a natural form of bloodletting. Their saliva contains a natural anti-coagulant that also anaesthetises the wound area, reducing pain from the bite of the leech. It was thought in medieval times that leeches only removed 'impure' blood from the body, leaving 'good' blood behind (see Source J). The use of leeches continued well beyond the medieval period. Indeed, demand for leeches in the nineteenth century was so high that they very nearly became extinct in the wild. They were used as an alternative to cupping and are still used in some procedures today.

> **THINK**
> 1. The barber surgeon in Source I is cutting hair and his assistant is washing hair. How can you tell from the image that he is a surgeon too?
> 2. Do you think Source J is an accurate image of a patient using leeches? How can you tell?
> 3. The *Régime du corps*, written by Aldobrandino of Siena (probably in 1285), was the first French published medical text book. Does that make it a reliable source for us?

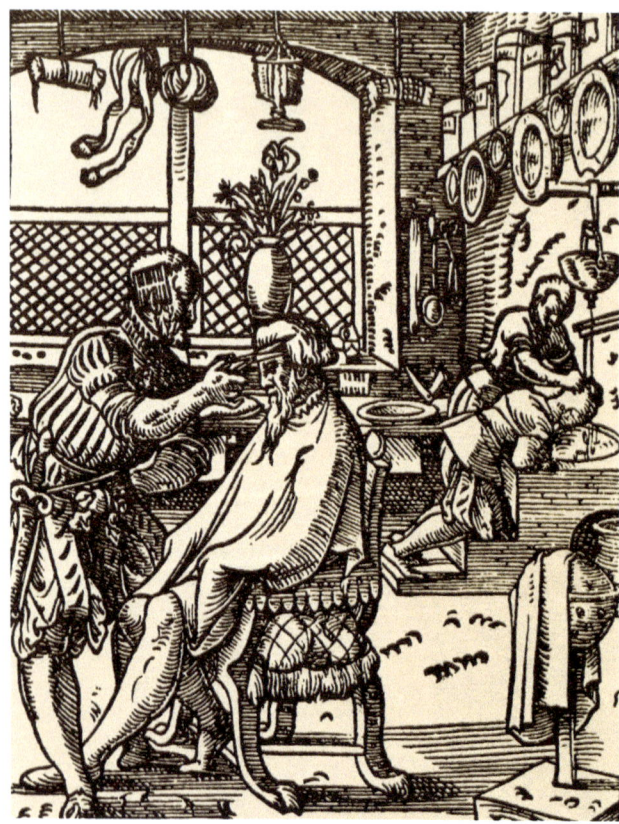

▲ Source I: Engraving of a barber-surgeon by Jost Amman, 1568

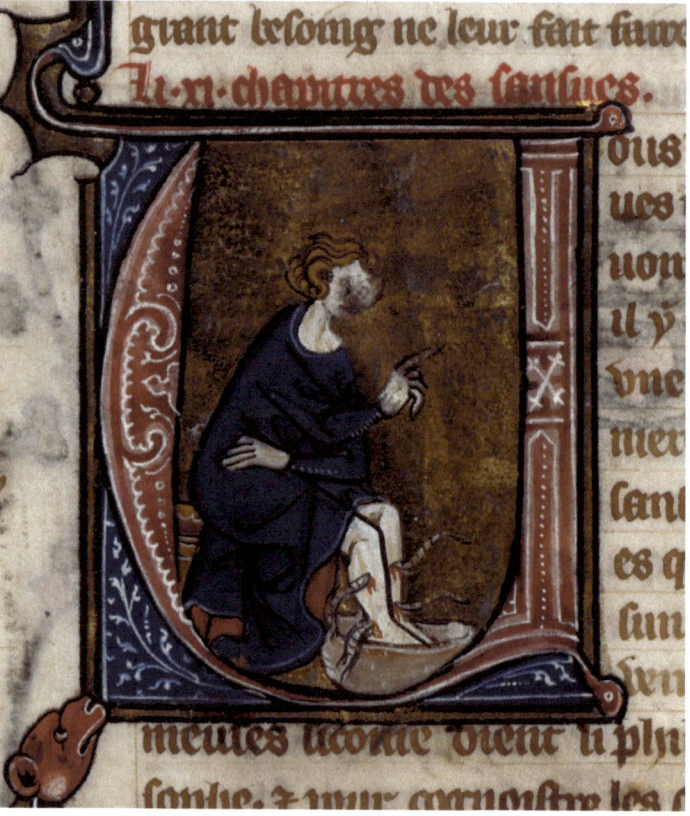

▲ Source J: Patient being treated with leeches, from the French medical treatise *Régime du corps*, published in 1256

Treatments in the early modern period

A lot of traditional treatments and remedies from the medieval era continued to be used in the early modern period but there were also some new developments.

'Ladies of the manor', such as Lady Johanna St John, played a role in healing in this period. As well as running a large household they would compile recipe books of cures (see Source K for one of her recipes).

> **Source K:** Lady Johanna St John's cure for a bleeding nose
>
> *A sheet of white paper, wett it in vinegar and dry it in an oven – when it is dry, wett it again and dry it as before, so doing 3 times, then make it into a powder and snuff up some of it into the nose, often, as well, when it does, and when it bleeds.*

During the early modern period some physicians wrote in English rather than Latin, in an attempt to help more people. Herbs were also used in a more coherent way than was previously the case by incorporating the doctrine of signatures (the idea that if a plant looked like a part of the body it could be used to treat that part of the body when it was ill) as well as astronomy.

New ingredients were also appearing from around the world. Rhubarb was hailed as a wonder-drug when it was first introduced from Asia. Tobacco was brought from North America by Walter Raleigh and, despite James I writing a famous book about the evils of tobacco, it quickly found many uses in herbal remedies. In fact there is a record of some schoolboys at Eton being beaten for refusing to smoke tobacco. Apparently smoking a pipe was regarded as an excellent way to keep the plague at bay!

The scientific approach to medicine, which involved observation, experiment and recording results, brought not just new ingredients for herbal medicines but new ideas on how to deal with disease too. New studies of mental illness, often referred to as 'melancholy', and other disciplines such as midwifery were also conducted during this period. Some individuals began to identify lifestyle issues such as taking fresh air and improving your diet as ways of preventing illness, rather than relying on doctors to cure them once they became ill.

> **THINK**
> 1 When would you rather have been ill – the medieval or early modern period?
> 2 Which treatments do you think were more effective, those of the medieval or early modern period? Why?

James Simpson and the development of anaesthetics

Surgery was accompanied by pain. Many surgeons believed patients *should* experience pain, as it helped them appreciate the efforts being made on their behalf. Copious amounts of alcohol or opium was often used to try to subdue a patient and thus make an operation easier to perform, although getting the right dose was very tricky. Sir Humphrey Davy was one of the first to use nitrous oxide, or laughing gas as we know it (see Source L). He invited his friends to inhale the gas from oiled silk bags. Quickly the gas was used as an anaesthetic to relieve pain during operations, but it was difficult to control the dose. In 1846 Robert Liston successfully amputated a leg using ether as an anaesthetic, copying his ideas from an American dentist, although one drawback of this was that sometimes the patient woke up in the middle of the operation!

In 1847 the Scottish scientist James Simpson (1811–70) used chloroform, after experimenting on himself and his friends, to reduce pain in childbirth. Chloroform induces dizziness, sleepiness and unconsciousness in patients, and needs to be carefully administered. Not surprisingly there was opposition in many quarters to the use of these painkillers, but this was partly overcome in 1853 when Queen Victoria used chloroform while having a baby. If it was good enough for the queen then it was good enough for anybody. All these painkillers had to be inhaled as a general anaesthetic in order to work. Finally, in the 1850s, coca leaves from South America were used to produce cocaine that could be used as a local anaesthetic – on the first occasion as drops in the eye. The use of cocaine rapidly spread, especially once it could be produced chemically after 1891. By the end of the century operations no longer had to be painful.

Anaesthetics did not necessarily make operations safer. As we have already seen, it was difficult to get the dose right with early painkillers. Also, surgeons tried more difficult operations because they could take longer to operate. But unfortunately, there was still no control over infection. Some surgeons had higher mortality rates using anaesthetics than before, so in the 1870s some stopped using chloroform altogether.

THINK

1. Why was pain seen to be a 'good thing' by surgeons?
2. To what extent does Source L show that anaesthetics did not necessarily make operations safer?
3. What part did science play in developing effective anaesthetics?
4. Why was it so difficult to get the dose right in early anaesthetics?
5. Humphrey Davy used nitrous oxide as a 'recreational drug', so why did the government recently (May 2016) ban the sale of nitrous oxide?

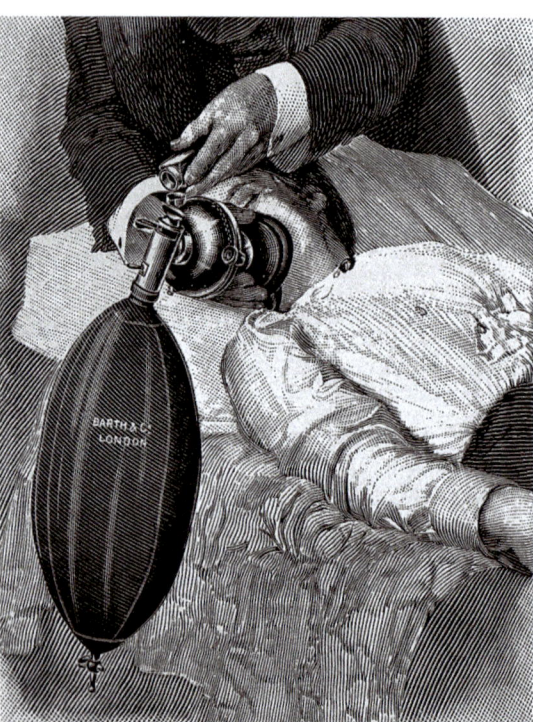

▲ **Source L:** Administering nitrous oxide and ether in the 1840s, as shown in a 1922 book on advances in medicine

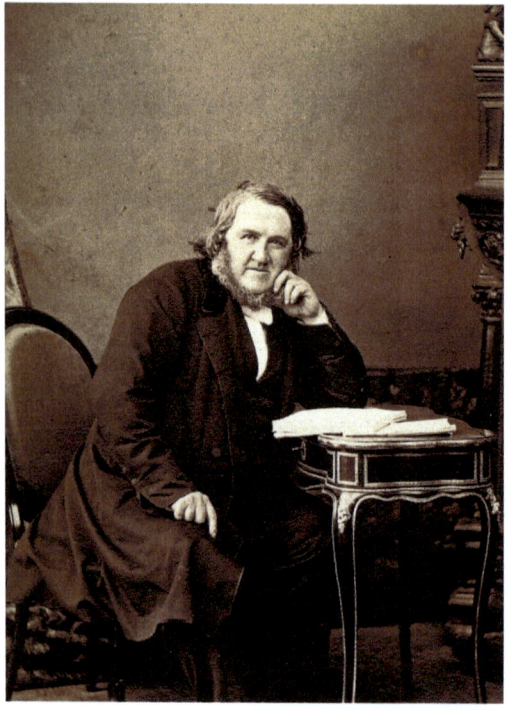

▲ James Simpson, photograph by Brigham

Joseph Lister and the use of antiseptics in the later nineteenth century

If we cut or graze ourselves today the first thing we do is wash the cut, then apply some antiseptic cream or a plaster. The idea is to prevent dirt getting into the wound, and to prevent infection. It is widely known that dirt and infection can kill. But all this is relatively recent. The biggest killer after surgery was sepsis, otherwise known as hospital gangrene, an infection caught during or after an operation. Surgeons completely opposed the idea that they themselves spread infection, through dirty clothes and unsterile equipment.

Ignaz Semmelweis was the pioneer in antiseptics in 1847. He was in charge of the maternity ward at Vienna General Hospital in Austria. He dramatically reduced the death rate on his maternity ward from around 35 per cent to less than 1 per cent by insisting that doctors wash their hands in calcium chloride solution before treating their patients. Despite publishing his results, very few other hospitals introduced the procedure.

Joseph Lister

Joseph Lister (1827–1912) was an English surgeon who, perhaps more than anybody, improved the chances of surviving surgery. After Pasteur published his germ theory (see page 59) Joseph Lister used an operating room sterilised with carbolic acid. He based his ideas on experiments he carried out on frogs. Frogs, as cold-blooded mammals, whose blood flowed more slowly, could be observed more clearly. Lister could see the impact of the changes he was introducing. His surgical instruments were sterilised with carbolic acid too. He also soaked the wound from time to time with carbolic acid, and used dressings sterilised in exactly the same way. Doing this he managed to reduce the mortality rate in his operations from 46 per cent to 15 per cent in only three years. In 1871 he invented a machine that sprayed carbolic acid over the entire room, surgeon, patient, assistants, everything. Others copied his methods and Lister became known as the 'Father of Antiseptic Surgery'.

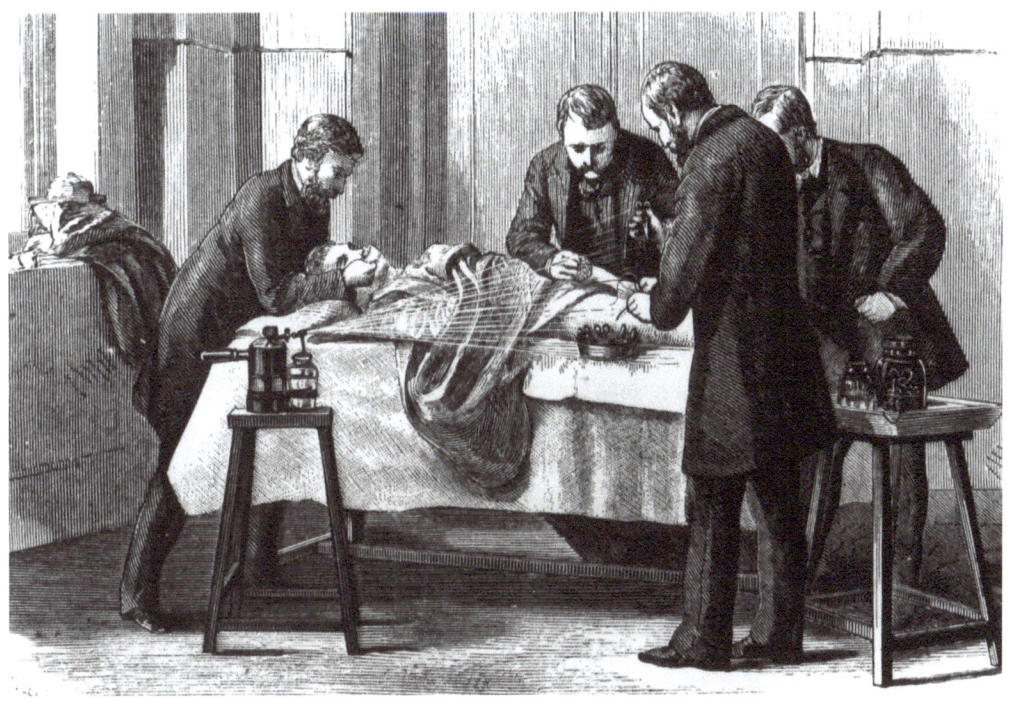

▲ **Source M:** An operation in progress using Lister's new carbolic spray

> **THINK**
>
> 1 Look at Source M. What what would it be like for (a) the patient, and (b) the medical staff, using this equipment?
> 2 In what ways is this an improvement on what went before Lister and antiseptic surgery?

Aseptic surgery: a real change at last?

Further improvements were made later in the century with the development of aseptic surgery. This followed on from the work of Robert Koch who discovered in 1878 that most disease was spread not by air but by contact with an infected surface. This led on to attempts to create a germ-free environment in which to carry out operations as a way of avoiding spreading infection.

In 1881 Charles Chamberland, a French biologist, invented a steam steriliser for medical instruments. He discovered that heating them in water at 140°C for 20 minutes completely sterilised them, making surgery much safer. This was the start of developing much simpler, less ornate and easier ways to sterilise tools for operations. As you might expect, few surgeons initially adopted this. The next step was by Gustav Neuber, a German surgeon in Kiel, who is recognised as having the first sterile operating theatre. He insisted on thorough scrubbing before staff entered the theatre; even the air in the room was sterilised. He published a paper on the process and his results in 1886 and this quickly set the standard for others to follow.

Surgical clothing

The final part of the battle against infection was the very gradual adoption of protective clothing – William Halsted in America started his team wearing surgical gloves because one of the nurses developed an allergic reaction on her hand to the carbolic spray they were using. He asked the Goodyear Rubber Company to make special thin rubber gloves for her to use. Berkeley Moyniham, a respected British surgeon working in Leeds, became the first in Britain to wear gloves for an operation, and later made a point of always changing his clothes for surgical gowns before entering an operating theatre. He was regarded by most surgeons as an oddity for doing so. In fact on one occasion his wife was presented with a bouquet made out of old rubber gloves.

> **Source N:** Berkeley Moyniham recalls his days as a student in Leeds in the 1880s
>
> *The surgeon arrived and threw off his jacket to avoid getting blood or pus on it. He rolled up his shirt sleeves and, in the corridor to the operation room, took an ancient frock from a cupboard; it bore signs of a chequered past, and was utterly stiff with old blood. One of these coats was worn with special pride, indeed joy, as it had belonged to a retired member of staff. The cuffs were rolled up to only just above the wrists, and the hands were washed in a sink. Once clean they were rinsed in carbolic-acid solution.*

THINK

1. What is the difference between antiseptic surgery and aseptic surgery?
2. Which in your opinion had the greater impact?
3. How had these new methods altered the approach of the surgeon training students at Leeds in the 1880s?
4. Consider Source N.
   - What impact has the move to antiseptic and aseptic surgery had on this surgeon?
   - What example is he setting his students?
   - This source was written down many years after the events it describes – does that affect its utility?

Twentieth-century developments

Marie Curie and the development of radiation

Marie Curie has been described as the most famous female scientist of all time (see Source O). She won the Nobel Prize in 1903 *and* in 1911. She is the only person to have won a Nobel Prize in both physics and chemistry, and was the first woman to win a Nobel Prize for science.

> **Source O:** Extract from an obituary for Marie Curie, *New York Times*, 1934
>
> *Few persons contributed more to the general welfare of mankind and to the advancement of science than the modest, self-effacing woman whom the world knew as Mme. Curie. Her epoch-making discoveries of polonium and radium, the subsequent honors that were bestowed upon her – she was the only person to receive two Nobel prizes – and the fortunes that could have been hers had she wanted them did not change her mode of life. She remained a worker in the cause of science, preferring her laboratory to a great social place in the sun.*

Marie Curie was born in Poland, and began work as a governess, as her father could not afford to pay for university. She was subsequently invited to live with her sister in Paris and was thus able eventually to attended university. She and her husband were the first to discover and isolate radium and polonium. These radioactive elements played a key role in destroying tissue, and thus opened up a way of treating cancer. Despite her husband being killed in a road accident in 1906, Marie continued to work – her 1911 Nobel Prize was for discovering a means to measure radiation. She also played a leading role in developing mobile X-ray units during the First World War, which could be used nearer the front line and thus making diagnosis and treatment of injured soldiers quicker and easier. She died in 1934, aged 67, from diseases brought on by excessive exposure to radiation.

> **THINK**
>
> 1. How useful is Source O in helping us understand Marie Curie's role in improving treatments of disease?
> 2. Look at Source P. What impression of Marie Curie and her work do you get from this image? Do you think it was posed? How useful is it to us in studying her work?

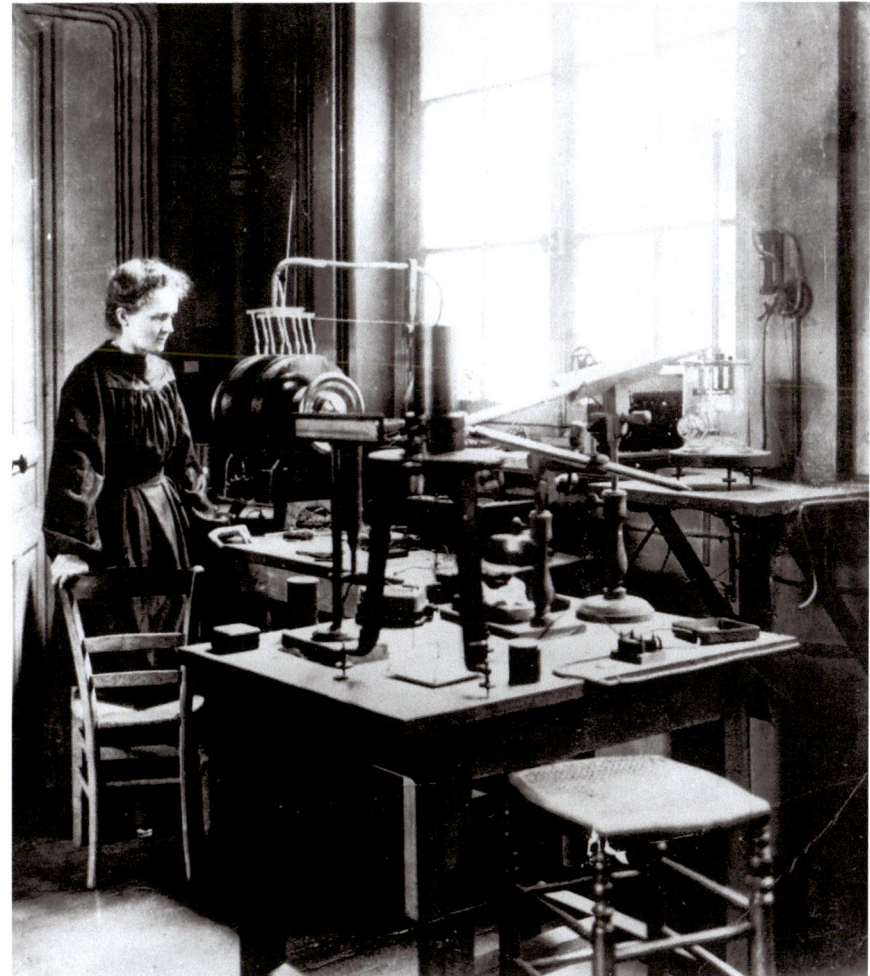

▲ **Source P:** Marie Curie in her laboratory

The roles of Fleming, Florey and Chain regarding antibiotics

Penicillin had been discovered in the nineteenth century. Indeed, Lister had used it once to treat infection in a wound, but had not published his notes. During the First World War Alexander Fleming observed that antiseptics seemed unable to prevent infection, especially in deep wounds. He decided to try to find something that would kill the microbes that caused infection. One of the most dangerous was staphylococci, which caused septicaemia. In 1928, on returning from holiday, he noticed a mould – penicillin – that had grown on one of his petri dishes. He also noticed that the staphylococci bacteria around the mould had been killed off. That was the start of the story of penicillin. He called it an antibiotic, meaning 'destructive of life'. Fleming published his results in 1929, but could not raise enough funds to develop the drug.

In 1937 Howard Florey and Ernst Chain, working at Oxford University, began to research penicillin after reading an article by Fleming. They overcame the difficulties of producing enough of the drug. They experimented first on mice, in 1940, and then on humans, in 1941. Their first trial, a policeman badly infected after being scratched by a rose bush, died after five days when their stock of the drug ran out, but the trial proved how effective penicillin was.

The Second World War provided a huge incentive to the development of the drug and in 1943 it was used for the first time on Allied troops in North Africa, with great success. America and Britain jointly produced huge quantities of penicillin and without doubt it saved many lives in 1944 and 1945. After the war it was widely used to treat many illnesses such as bronchitis, impetigo, pneumonia, tonsillitis, syphilis, meningitis, boils, abscesses and many other kinds of wounds. Fleming, Chain and Florey received the Nobel Prize for Medicine in 1945. Other antibiotics followed, such as streptomycin in 1944; tetracycline in 1953; and mitomycin in 1956.

ALEXANDER FLEMING, 1881–1955

- Trained as a doctor and served in the Army Medical Corps during the First World War.
- He became professor of his medical school in 1928 and published many papers on bacteriology, immunology and chemotherapy.
- He was knighted for his work in 1944.
- He was jointly awarded the Nobel Prize in 1945 for his work on penicillin.

THINK

1. What part did chance play in the discovery of penicillin?
2. What part did war play in the development of penicillin?
3. Who, in your opinion, deserves the title, 'Father of Penicillin'? Why?
4. What does Source Q tell us about the chances of wounded soldiers recovering (a) during the Second World War, and (b) during the First World War?

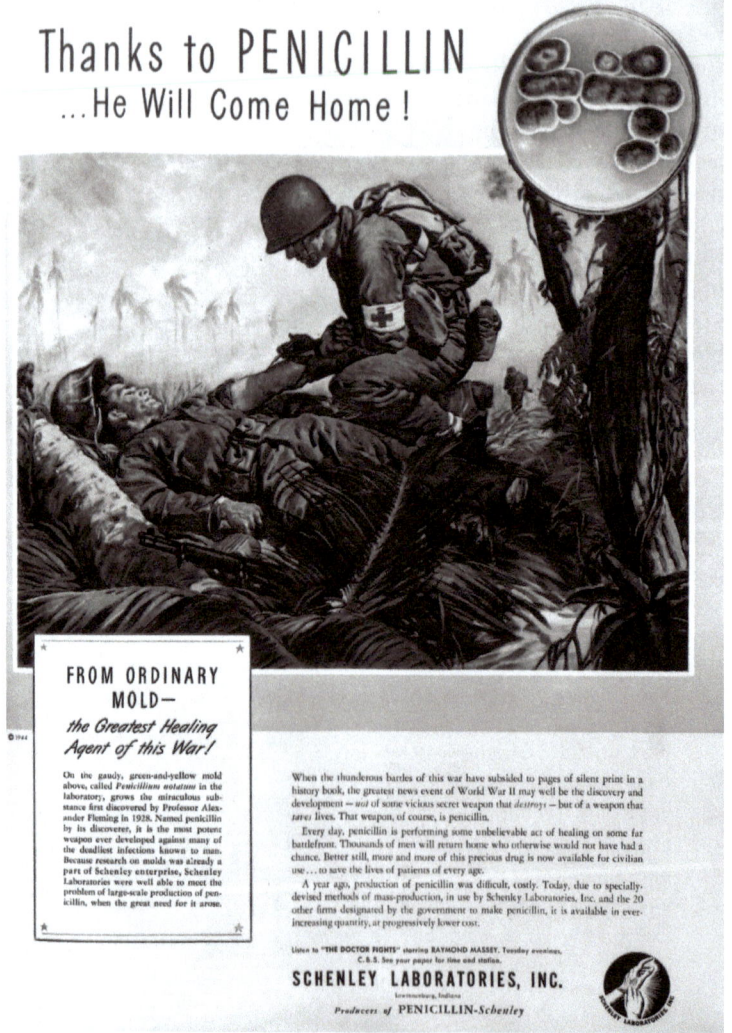

▲ **Source Q:** An advert for penicillin, 1945

Dr Christian Barnard and transplant surgery

The earlier part of this chapter will have shown you that there have been huge changes in the way surgery is carried out, and in its success rates. There have also been major changes in the *types* of surgery undertaken. The year 1952 saw the first kidney transplant. In 1961 the first British implanted heart pacemaker – an electrical device that keeps the heart pumping blood around the body – was developed, along with heart bypass surgery. In 1967 the world's first heart transplant operation was undertaken in Cape Town, South Africa, by Dr Christian Barnard. His patient lived for 18 days. There were two main problems – the availability of replacement organs (still a major problem today) and rejection of the transplant. This has been largely solved by the development of immunosupressive drugs, such as cyclosporine, which help the body accept the replacement organ. Now, transplants are routine with nearly 181 heart transplants having taken place in England in 2014 alone.

Hip replacements (replacing worn-out joints with new artificial ones) were introduced in 1972, bringing mobility to many who previously had found walking difficult. Out of date? Keyhole surgery is now commonplace, reducing the intrusiveness of operating on someone. There are even robotic operation systems licensed in the USA. Mortality rates from operations are carefully monitored and there are even 'league tables' for hospitals and surgeons so patients can choose the 'best' place for their treatment.

Modern advances in cancer treatment and surgery

Following on from the pioneering work of Marie Curie, throughout much of the twentieth century radiation therapy has been used to treat cancerous cells, becoming more and more refined and easier to target as technology has improved the technique. This has been supplemented by chemotherapy, the use of powerful drugs to kill cancerous cells. This has become more widespread since the Second World War and is often used for cancerous cells that are out of reach of surgery. Encouraging results have followed from a combination of surgery or radiation therapy and chemotherapy. Cancer is still a major killer, but more and more types of cancer are either being cured or controlled by these treatments. The key to success is often early diagnosis.

Finally, surgery is also used to remove cancerous growths. Mastectomy (removal of a woman's breast) or lung transplants are perhaps the most common forms of surgery used today to fight cancer. Surgery is always viewed as something of a gamble, as it is quite common for the cancer to return even after successful surgery to remove the infected tissue. In earlier times surgery was often required to find out if a patient had cancer. Now, with scanning techniques and fibre-optic micro cameras, it is possible to 'see' inside a patient's body without major surgery, thus reducing the impact of diagnosis.

> **ACTIVITY**
>
> Working with a partner, prepare a debate to argue which of the advances in surgery in the twentieth century mentioned on this page had the biggest impact on illness and disease.

> **THINK**
> 1. Why was it so difficult at first to successfully transplant organs?
> 2. How have these difficulties been overcome?
> 3. It is ethical to use the body parts of one person to keep another person alive?

Alternative treatments: what if you could not afford to see the doctor?

We have seen throughout this book that many people either *chose not* to visit a medical professional, or *could not* afford to. They relied on family remedies, or the local 'wise woman' to treat them. This hadn't changed for the first half of the twentieth century at least, as Source R shows.

A growing belief in alternative medicine

Controversies like the thalidomide case, where a medicine prescribed for morning sickness and nausea in pregnant women caused babies to be born with missing limbs, made some people distrust orthodox medicine, and there has been a huge increase in interest in what became known as alternative or holistic medicine. Treatments such as hydrotherapy, aromatherapy, hypnotherapy and acupuncture became popular in some quarters. Many of them were based on old, traditional treatments using herbs and 'pure' treatments designed to work in harmony with the body, rather than as a chemical barrage against illness. Nearly every high street now includes a health food shop where a wide range of alternative herbal remedies are freely available to buy. Acupuncture, for example, is a traditional Chinese method of treating illness by sticking needles into various parts of the body and tapping into the natural flows of energy around the body. Prince Charles has long been a supporter of homeopathy, claiming, in a speech to the World Health Organization in Geneva in 2006, that it is 'rooted in ancient traditions that intuitively understood the need to maintain balance and harmony with our minds, bodies and the natural world'.

Not everyone agrees. The British Medical Association has described homeopathy as 'witchcraft' and the government's chief scientific adviser dismissed it as 'nonsense'. The evidence appears conflicting, but nevertheless alternative medicine has a strong hold on many people who dislike the idea of filling one's body with chemicals.

> **Source R:** From an interview with Kathleen Davys, who lived in Birmingham. She was one of 13 children. The local doctor charged sixpence a visit – and that was before paying for any treatment or medicine
>
> *Headaches, we had vinegar and brown paper, for whooping cough we had camphorated oil rubbed on our chests, or goose fat. For mumps we had stockings round our throats and for measles we had tea stewed in the teapot by the fire – all different kinds of home cures. They thought they were better than going to the doctor's. Well, they couldn't afford the doctor because sixpence in those days was like looking at a £5 note today.*

ACTIVITY

Discuss with an older relative about home cures, or do some research into home remedies to find out what people did in the recent past.

THINK

1. You might remember the nursery rhyme 'Jack and Jill'. Jack went to bed to mend his head with vinegar and brown paper. Does this mean nursery rhymes can be a useful source of evidence for knowledge about medicine?
2. What are the similarities between Figure 3.1 and the Ancient Greek theory of the four humours?

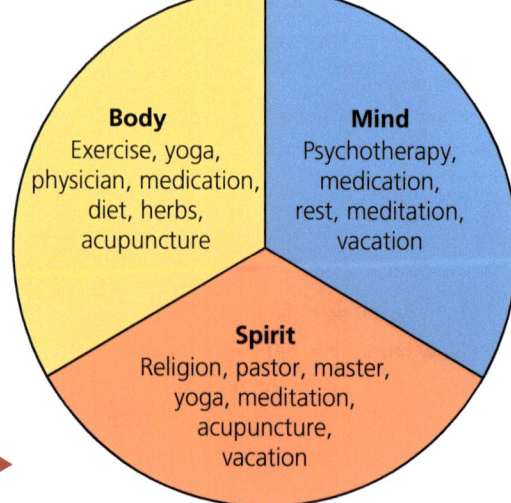

Figure 3.1: How one organisation promotes holistic medicine

3 Attempts to treat and cure illness and disease

FOCUS TASK REVISITED

1 Having worked through this chapter carefully you should now have a note of each cure for an illness you have come across, in your copy of the table below.

Illness or disease	Cure	Effectiveness at the time	Effectiveness today
Headache	Drink camomile tea and lie down	5	5

2 Fill in the final two columns, giving the cure a rating for effectiveness (1 = low, 5 = high), both for how people at the time thought of it as a cure, and how you, today, rank it as a cure.
3 What can you deduce about attempts to treat and cure illness and disease from your completed table?
4 Now you have explored causes of illness, attempts at prevention and attempts to cure illness, when do you think was the best time to be ill? Why?

ACTIVITIES

1 Draw a spider diagram showing attempts to treat and cure illness. You have your table from the focus task, which should now list all the illnesses and cures you have come across in this chapter.
2 How do they link together? Is there a direct link between medieval herbalists and alternative medicine today? Or between the more scientific approach of the early modern period and the twentieth century? And how are you going to show these links? Your diagram might look something like this:

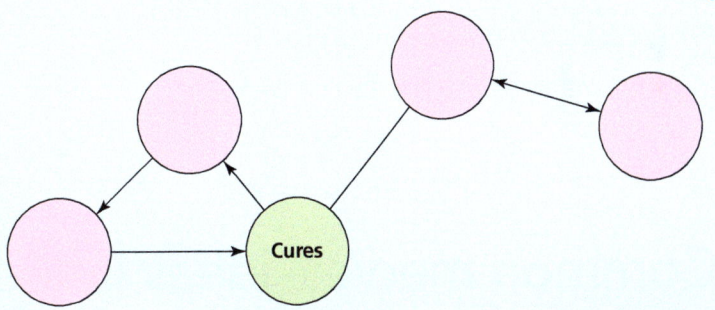

TOPIC SUMMARY

- Some early herbal treatments were surprisingly effective.
- The scientific approach, based on observation, experimentation and measuring, ushered in great changes to the treatment of disease.
- The effective use of anaesthetics and antiseptic made surviving surgery much more likely.
- Technology and discoveries have transformed treatment of disease in the twentieth century.
- Some people prefer to rely on non-invasive 'natural' medicine to treat illnesses.
- Apothecaries and barber-surgeons were surprisingly effective at treating some illnesses and diseases.
- Great efforts were made to make surgery and surgeons cleaner – although not all surgeons appreciated this.
- Transplants are now increasingly common, and very successful ways to treat disease.
- However, many changes only helped people if they could afford to visit the doctor.
- Some diseases have been conquered, but others remain a problem for society.

Practice questions

1 Study Source K and Source J. Which of the two sources is the more useful to a historian studying attempts to cure illnesses in medieval and early modern times? *(For guidance, see page 123.)*
2 Describe the development and use of antiseptics in the nineteenth century. *(For guidance, see page 125.)*
3 Explain why the development of antibiotics was important in the cure of illness and disease in the twentieth century. *(For guidance, see page 126.)*
4 Outline how attempts to treat illness and disease have changed over the last 1000 years. *(For guidance, see page 127.)*

4 Advances in medical knowledge

This chapter focuses on the key question: How much progress has been made in medical knowledge over time?

It is easy to assume that medical knowledge in medieval times was limited, yet there is plenty of evidence of successful medical treatment, if you had access to a doctor, even from the Stone Age. It was perhaps the Renaissance, and the later arrival of scientific method, that really changed our understanding of illness and made significant advances in medical knowledge, something that continues apace today. This chapter explores many of the 'turning points' in the growth of medical knowledge.

FOCUS TASK

1. For each section of this chapter, we would like you to decide what progress has been made in medical knowledge, and then to try to measure 'how much'. Each section will have a card like this:

Complete the card as you work through the section.

Breakthrough:	To what extent [1–5]
Galen	2
....	....
....	....

Common medical ideas in the medieval period

Where did medieval ideas about health come from? People have always known how to look after themselves. There is clear evidence of successful operations carried out with flint tools in the Stone Age. Archaeological evidence showed that some of these patients survived. The Indus Valley civilisation was well aware of the importance of clean running water and sewers. There is even a structure identified as a huge Public Bath house in Mohen Daro, dating from around 2500 BC. Pharaohs in Ancient Egypt had their court physicians, and we know about some of their medical practices from papyrus records recovered from tombs. The Greeks had asclepions, or places of healing, that were temples to Asclepius, the god of healing. The Romans went to great lengths to bring fresh water to their towns and cities. Their bath-houses and underfloor heating can be found in most Roman towns, for example, Vindolanda in Northumberland. Bald's *Leechbook* is an Anglo-Saxon medical text full of remedies and medicines, some of which modern medical research has shown worked.

Yet much of this medical knowledge seems to have been 'lost' during the so-called 'Dark Ages,' after the Romans left. Muslim writers, such as Ibn Sīnā, played a very important role in saving much of this lost knowledge, translating the works of Ancient Greece and Rome into Arabic, that eventually passed on to Western Europe. At this time there is no doubt that Arabic medicine was much in advance of that in Western Europe.

THINK

What, according to Source A, were the main differences between Muslim and European medicine?

Source A: An account written by a Muslim doctor Usama ibn Munqidh, *c.*1175

They brought to me a knight with a sore on his leg; and a woman who was feeble-minded. To the knight I applied a small *poultice*; and the woman I put on diet to turn her humour wet. Then a French doctor came and said, 'This man knows nothing about treating them.' He then said, 'Bring me a sharp axe.' Then the doctor laid the leg of the knight on a block of wood and told a man to cut off the leg with the axe, upon which the marrow flowed out and the patient died on the spot. He then examined the woman and said, 'There is a devil in her head.' He therefore took a razor, made a deep cross-shaped cut on her head, peeled away the skin until the bone of the skull was exposed, and rubbed it with salt. The woman also died instantly.

Hippocrates, Galen and the four humours

Perhaps two men, more than any others, contributed to the Western view of medicine at this time. These were Hippocrates and Galen. We have already come across Hippocrates, 'the father of modern medicine', in Chapter 2. New doctors around the world still take the Hippocratic Oath when they start to practise. Altogether there are around 60 texts remaining that are attributed to Hippocrates, although many may have been written by his followers.

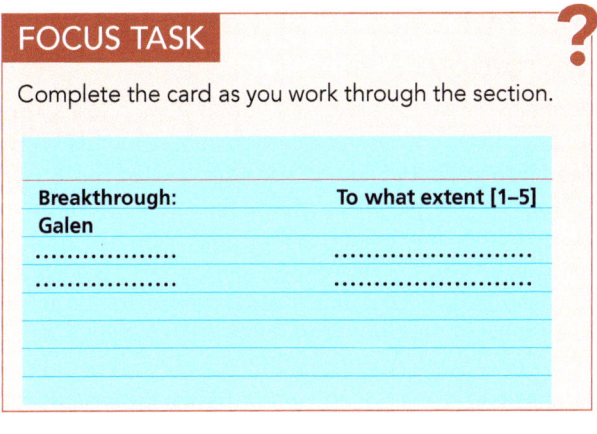

> **FOCUS TASK**
>
> Complete the card as you work through the section.
>
> | Breakthrough: Galen | To what extent [1–5] |
> | --- | --- |
> | .... | .... |
> | .... | .... |

Galen was born in what is now Turkey in AD130. He studied medicine in Egypt before moving to Rome. He followed the ideas of Hippocrates, but was able to take them further. Although prevented from practising on people, he believed dissection was the best way to discover the secret workings of the human body. Despite being only able to dissect animals, he developed a better practical knowledge of how the human body worked. Three years working as a doctor in a gladiator school gave him plenty of opportunity to further improve his knowledge and techniques. Galen also placed great emphasis on listening to a patient's pulse as a diagnostic tool – a technique still widely used today.

Galen's work arrived in Europe via Islamic texts and beliefs. Greek translations were made in Salerno, in Italy (the first medical university dating from around AD900), and rapidly became accepted as university medical texts. Church leaders looked carefully at Galen's works and decided that they fitted with Christian ideas because throughout he referred to 'the Creator'. Doctors believed his ideas were correct and that it was nearly impossible to improve his work. As Salerno was a common stopping-off point en route to the Holy Land, Galen's ideas rapidly spread throughout Europe and became accepted as medical orthodoxy.

The four humours

Key to both Hippocrates and Galen's medical knowledge was the theory of the **four humours**. Hippocrates wrote:

> The human body contains blood, phlegm, yellow bile and black bile. These are the things that make up its constitution and cause its pains and health. Health is primarily that state in which these constituent substances are in the correct proportion to each other, both in strength and quantity, and are well mixed. Pain occurs when one of the substances presents either a deficiency or an excess, or is separated in the body and not mixed with others.

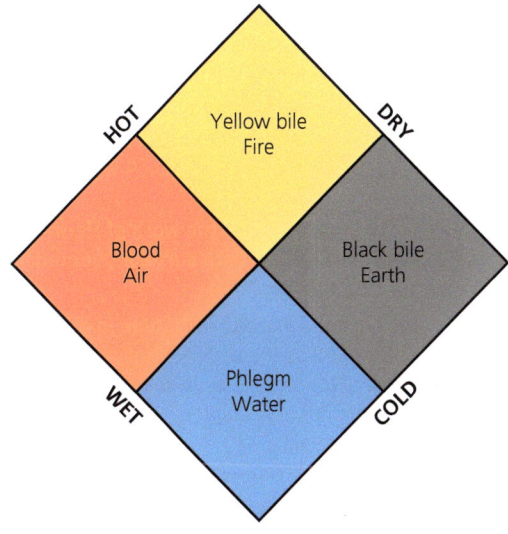

Figure 4.1: The four humours

So to remain healthy a body needed to keep the four humours in balance. As you can see from Figure 4.1, some humours are 'hot' and therefore create sweating illnesses; and some humours are 'cold', creating illnesses such as melancholia.

Different foods and different seasons could affect the humours, so it was important to do all things in moderation to keep the body in balance. During the medieval period much of the medical knowledge was based on the idea of the four humours and keeping them in balance. It was only later, during the Renaissance, that people began to challenge the work of Galen, and develop new medical knowledge.

> **ACTIVITIES**
>
> 1. Use the internet to research Hippocrates and Galen. You might like to consider the following questions:
>   - ☐ Where did their ideas about medicine come from?
>   - ☐ How did these ideas reach the Muslim world?
>   - ☐ How did their ideas then reach Europe and Britain?
>   - ☐ How influential were these ideas in shaping medical knowledge in Britain in the medieval period and later?

The influence of alchemy and astrology

Alchemy, as we have seen in Chapter 2, was closely linked to science, and to the search to turn base metals such as lead into gold. Alchemists also searched for the 'Elixir of Life' so that people could live forever. Many of them were monks or priests who were often the best educated people. Much of their work had an impact on science and medical knowledge. Alchemists were the first to produce hydrochloric acid and nitric acid; they identified new elements such as antimony and arsenic, and paved the way for the new science of chemistry. Some of the equipment they developed is still in use today.

Doctors believed that the movement of the stars influenced the personalities of people and the inner workings of the human body. Hence, to be successful, you needed to study the stars. By the end of the 1500s, physicians in many countries of Europe were required by law to calculate the position of the moon before carrying out complicated medical procedures, such as surgery or bleeding. Each part of the body was associated with an astrological sign. Medicines could only be effective if the plants were collected at the right cycle of the moon. Medicines and surgery were only safe at the correct time of the month (see Source B).

> **Source B:** An extract from the work of Henri de Mondeville, a thirteenth-century French surgeon, quoted in Nathan Belofsky, *Strange Medicine*
>
> *The humours are agitated at that time [a full moon]. The brain waxes in the skull as the water raises in the river ... thus the membranes of the skull rise up and consequently come nearer to the skull, so that they could be more easily damaged by surgical instruments.*

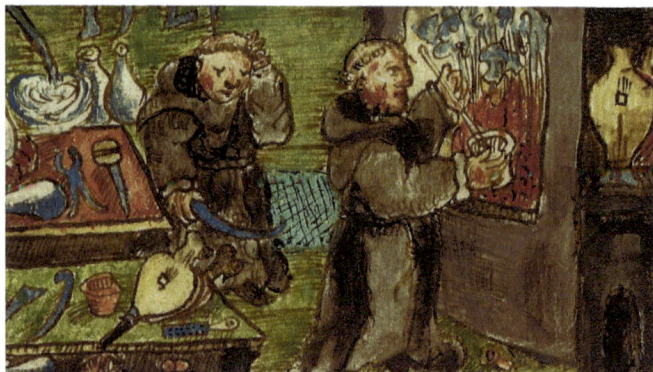

▲ **Source C:** From a medieval manuscript showing two monks in their laboratory

The role of the church in developing medical knowledge

The church was central to most peoples' lives in medieval times, so its attitude to medicine would have a profound influence on medical progress and developments. Most importantly, the church encouraged people to pray for deliverance from illness, for forgiveness of their sins, and to prepare for the afterlife. (Remember, most surgery was extremely dangerous.) As well as prayer, offerings could buy **indulgences**, and going on a pilgrimage to a holy shrine might bring about a cure. Pilgrims would often leave a miniature copy of the infected body part at the shrine, and hope that prayer and belief would indeed bring about a cure.

The church set up university schools of medicine throughout Europe where physicians could be trained using the texts of Hippocrates and Galen. It might take ten years to train as a physician. In fact it was often through these university schools and in monasteries that the old texts were hand copied by monks and thus survived. Many of them arrived in the West in Arabic translation (see page 54). Most studies of dissection were still based on Galen's writings and his work on dissection was based on working on animals. Therefore the church's insistence on using Galen and his works widely limited progress in understanding the workings of the human body. Scientists who tried to insist on scientific method and observation often ran into difficulty. Roger Bacon, a Franciscan monk and lecturer at Oxford University, was arrested around 1277 for spreading anti-church views.

> **THINK**
> 1. Do you think astrology and alchemy helped or hindered advances in medical knowledge at the time?
> 2. Why were science and alchemy so closely linked in medieval times?
> 3. How did the church help advances in medical knowledge?
> 4. Look at Source C. What do you think these monks might be doing? Do you think the artist has been into a laboratory? How can you tell?
> 5. How useful is Source C in helping us understand the part played by (a) alchemy and (b) the church in advances in medical knowledge?

The influence of the medical work of Vesalius, Paré and Harvey in the sixteenth and seventeenth centuries

The Renaissance and Galen

Initially, the Renaissance led to a revival of all things ancient. Many of Galen's works were re-translated from Arabic into Greek and Latin. Texts were compared and efforts made to get back to the original meaning. By 1525 his complete works had been published in Greek and translations into Latin soon followed. Galen was regarded as the font of all medical knowledge, to be slavishly copied.

Galen's position was soon to be challenged. The very essence of the Renaissance was to question things. And the more artists and surgeons studied anatomy, and the more humans they dissected, the more they began to notice discrepancies between what Galen said and what they were discovering for themselves. The initial reaction was that Galen was right and the current anatomists were wrong. But gradually enough opinion grew to successfully challenge Galen and cast doubts on his observations. Once challenged on anatomy, other challenges followed. The medical world seemed to be split into two, depending on how strongly you supported Galen. It also seemed to split into two between physicians, who mostly learned from texts and lectures and thus largely supported Galen's ideas; and surgeons, who were exploring the human body on a daily basis and were learning by experimenting and experience. Scientific discovery played a part in this as new tools, like the microscope, allowed both scientists and medical men to look at things in ever more detail. But so too did William Caxton and his printing press, which allowed the much more rapid spread of ideas from 1476 onwards.

Vesalius and anatomy

Andreas Vesalius (1514–64) was born in Brussels but studied medicine in Paris and Padua in Italy. He was appointed professor of surgery and anatomy in Padua. Perhaps most importantly he carried out his own dissections and firmly believed anatomy was the key to understanding how the human body worked. In 1543 he published *De humani corporis fabrica libri septem*, which completely changed attitudes to medicine. Vesalius challenged Galen's works on human anatomy, and developed much more accurate views of the inside of the human body by, unlike Galen, looking at and dissecting humans rather than animals. His work was very influential for early modern medicine both because it gave doctors more detailed knowledge of human anatomy and because it encouraged them to investigate critically the claims of ancient medical authorities.

> **FOCUS TASK**
>
> Complete the card as you work through the section.
>
> | Breakthrough: Vesalius | To what extent [1–5] |
> |---|---|
> | .... | .... |
> | .... | .... |

Paré and treating wounds

Ambroise Paré (1510-90) began his medical work as an apprentice to his elder brother, a barber-surgeon. He is perhaps the most famous example from the sixteenth century of someone who adopted the new scientific ways of treating disease. He trained at the Hotel du Dieu hospital in Paris before becoming a surgeon in the French army for 30 years. At the siege of Milan in 1536 he ran out of hot oil for cauterising wounds. He made up a mixture of egg yolk, turpentine and oil of roses to dress raw wounds – much less painful and, as he discovered the next morning, much more effective at encouraging healing. He also used ligatures to tie-off wounds after amputation – again instead of cauterisation – and found that wounds healed better. Later he helped develop artificial limbs for those who had lost a hand or a leg due to their wounds. His time as an army surgeon allowed Paré to observe his patients and treat them more effectively. He published his experiences in a book, *Les oeuvres* in 1575, and became famous across Europe. He is considered one of the fathers of modern surgery.

> **THINK**
>
> 1. What changes did the Renaissance bring to medical knowledge?
> 2. Who do you think had the greater impact – Vesalius or Paré?
> 3. What do you think helped bring about change more – war or science and technology?

William Harvey and the circulation of blood

Harvey's most famous work, *On the Motion of the Heart*, was published in 1628. It, more than any other book at the time, challenged the work of Galen and the Ancients, and changed medicine for ever.

While studying in Padua, Harvey was taught that the veins in the human body had valves, and blood pumped only one way. But no one understood how or why. Later in his career Harvey experimented on animals, and it was during this experimentation that he discovered blood was pumped around the body in a circular motion. This led to his famous discovery of the circulation of the blood.

His discovery was made partly as a result of theoretical work – he was unable to see the tiny capillaries which are the smallest blood vessels – but also as a result of experiment and observation. His work on cold-blooded amphibians, whose blood circulates much more slowly, allowed him to see blood pumping around the body and his most famous experiment, described in his book, showed blood moving in a patient's forearm. With this experiment he was able to show convincingly that the heart worked as a pump, and that blood flowed in a 'one-way system' around the human body.

He was also able to show that Galen's belief that the liver, not the heart, was the centre of the human body, was completely wrong. Galen also believed that the liver made new blood to replace that lost around the body. Harvey's work on the circulation of blood around the body proved that this was wrong, and also challenged the idea of 'bleeding' as a cure – if Harvey was right then it was impossible for the body to have too much blood.

How was Harvey's work greeted by contemporaries?

As you might imagine, those who supported Galen totally rejected Harvey's work. They argued that Harvey could not see capillaries and therefore could not prove their existence – it was another 60 years before capillaries were observed in action. Some refused to accept the role of experiments in challenging the ancient texts. Many were very conservative and resistant to change. In fact Harvey himself told a friend that he lost many patients after 1628 because of his 'crack-pot ideas'.

WILLIAM HARVEY

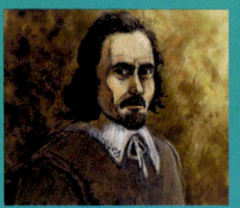

- Born in Kent in 1578 and educated at Cambridge University.
- Studied medicine at the University of Padua in Italy.
- Returned to England in 1602 and set himself up as a physician. His career benefited from his marriage to the daughter of Elizabeth I's physician.
- Accepted a post at St Bartholomew's Hospital in 1609 and worked there for the rest of his life. Appointed physician to both James I and Charles I.

THINK

1. How was William Harvey able to prove that blood circulated around the human body?
2. Why did people oppose his work?
3. What does the story of William Harvey tell us about medical knowledge in the seventeenth century?
4. Is it fair to say that William Harvey's work changed medicine for ever?

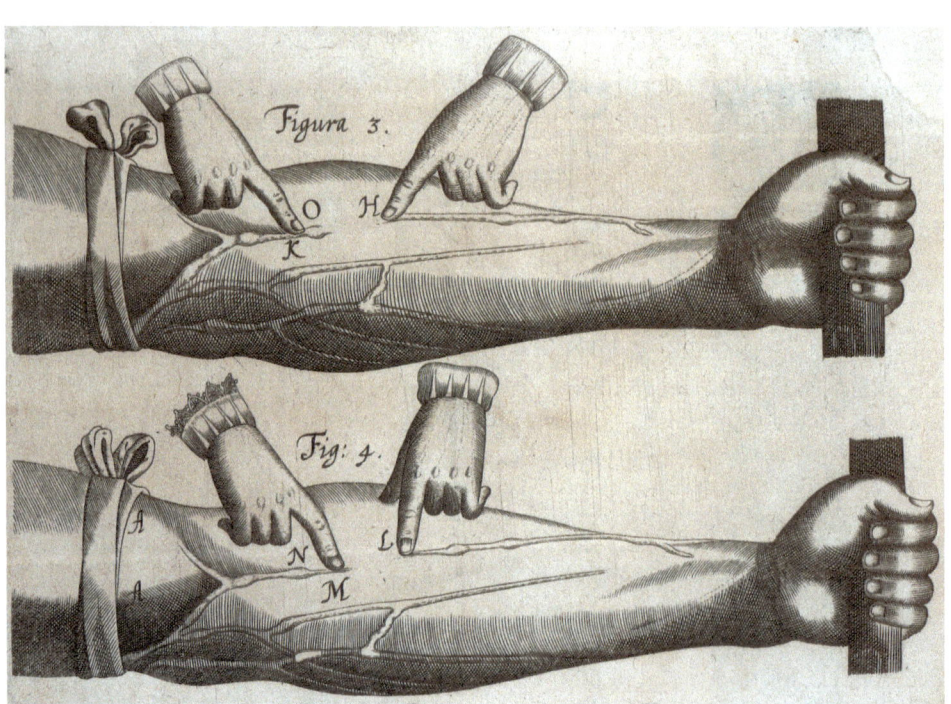

▲ **Source D:** From *Exercitatio anatomica de motu cordis et sanguinis in animalibus*, by William Harvey, 1628, showing how blood circulates through the veins

Nineteenth century advances in medical knowledge: improved knowledge of the germ theory

Pasteur and Koch

At the beginning of the nineteenth century most people still believed ill-health was caused by bad air, the 'spontaneous combustion' of disease or an imbalance of the four humours. Germ theory changed all that. As we have seen in Chapter 2 (page 40), by the 1880s and 1890s huge steps had been taken in identifying the cause of disease, thus enabling techniques to be developed to effectively treat illnesses.

Three people played a major part in this breakthrough: Pasteur, Koch and Ehrlich. They were not the only ones, but they led the way in experimental science. Louis Pasteur was the first person to establish the link between germs and disease. He argued that micro-organisms were responsible for disease, and that if only we could discover these micro-organisms then a vaccine could be developed to specifically target the disease. This allowed him to develop effective vaccines to target specific diseases. His first work was on chicken cholera and this led in 1880 to an effective vaccine against rabies.

Robert Koch took this work further. In the laboratory he was able to link particular germs to particular diseases, in effect developing the new science of bacteriology. In 1882 he identified the specific bacillus that caused tuberculosis and in 1883 and 1884 those responsible for cholera, thus confirming the work of John Snow in Britain in 1854 (see Chapter 2, page 35). Following this, he and his students rapidly isolated the causes of many diseases including diphtheria, typhoid, pneumonia, plague, tetanus and whooping cough, all of which were major killer diseases in Britain. He and his team also developed a technique for using dyes to stain bacteria to make it easier to see and study them under a microscope. His work was regarded as so important he was awarded a Nobel Prize in 1905.

Paul Ehrlich

Paul Ehrlich, a German physician and scientist, was one of Koch's students. He epitomises the scientific approach to identifying and treating diseases. He is perhaps best known for Salvarsan 606, developed in 1910, the first effective treatment for syphilis, a sexually transmitted disease (STD), which at the time was widespread. It was called '606' because it was literally the 606th drug he and his colleagues had used to try to kill the germs causing syphilis. Salvarsan 606 was the first of what became known as 'magic bullets', carefully designed drugs targeting the specific germs causing that illness and having little or no effect on any other part of the human body. No wonder people were so excited about the power of science to eradicate disease.

The impact of germ theory

Germ theory completely changed medical knowledge about the causes of diseases and how to treat them. It came about through careful scientific observation and experiment, and established once and for all the link between bacteria and disease.

> **FOCUS TASK**
>
> Complete the card as you work through this section.
>
> | Breakthrough: | To what extent [1–5] |
> |---|---|
> | Pasteur | |
> | .... | .... |
> | .... | .... |

> **THINK**
> 1. In what ways did germ theory change medical knowledge?
> 2. Did Koch deserve a Nobel Prize?

The development of scanning techniques in the twentieth century: X-rays, ultrasound and MRI scans

FOCUS TASK

Complete the card as you work through the section.

Breakthrough: X-rays	To what extent [1–5]
....	....
....	....

The development of scanning techniques has revolutionised medical knowledge, especially in the last 30 years or so. Safe, non-invasive technology allows medical staff to identify disease earlier; understand better how diseases affect and spread through the body; and improve medical care.

X-rays

X-rays were discovered by Wilhelm Röntgen, a German scientist, in 1895, building on work by other scientists. He found that radiation would pass through the body at different rates, depending on whether it encountered bones or flesh. He realised he could photograph bones and his discovery rapidly led to the use of X-rays to investigate broken bones. Initial doses of radiation were high, leading to severe side-effects.

During the First World War mobile X-ray units were set up to check for bullets, shrapnel and other 'foreign bodies' inside wounded soldiers' bodies, thus allowing quicker and safer surgery, saving many lives (see Source E). Since the war, X-rays have been routinely used in hospitals to investigate problems with bones and teeth (see Source F).

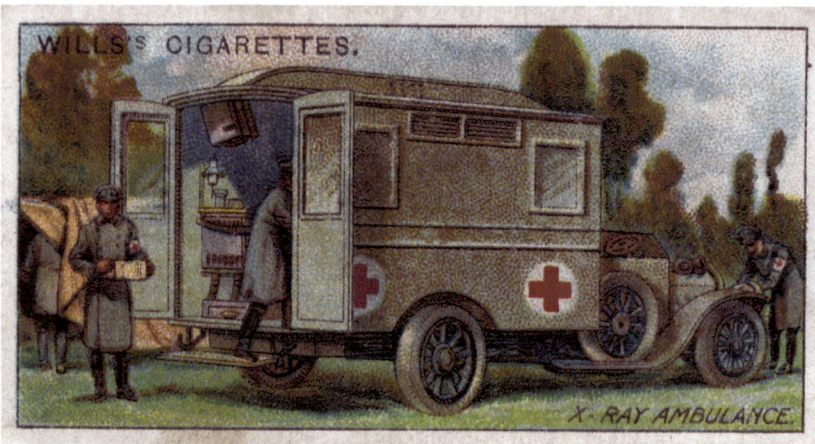

▲ **Source E:** A cigarette card from the First World War showing a French mobile X-ray van

THINK

1. Why was the development of X-ray technology so helpful in advancing medical knowledge?
2. Which is more useful to us in understanding the impact of X-rays, Source E or Source F? Why?

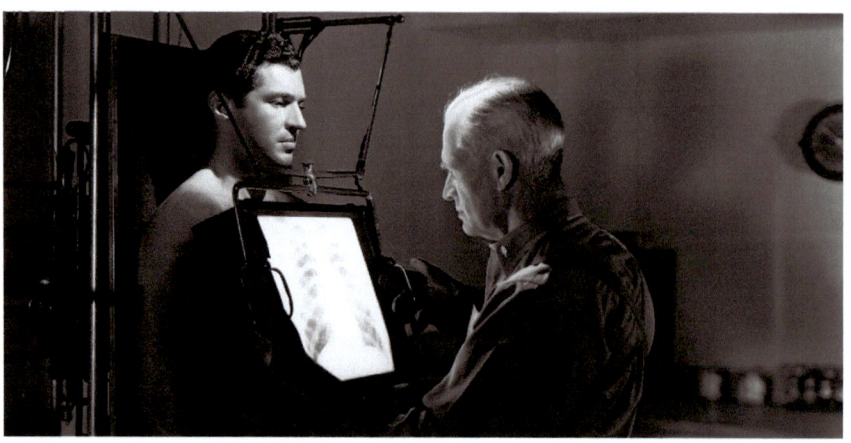

▲ **Source F:** A doctor examining a patient using X-ray equipment

Ultrasound

During the Second World War sound waves were used to detect German submarines. The British called this system ASDIC while the Americans referred to it as Sonar. It was after the war that it was realised you could use sound to 'see' inside the human body, by using high frequency sound waves. This avoided the need to use radiation, as in X-rays. It also produced 3D images. Ultrasound is used for images of organs in the body, such as the heart, liver and muscles, rather than bones, thus complementing X-rays. It is also, since the 1970s, routinely used to check the progress of unborn babies, to see if they are growing normally.

MRI

MRI (magnetic resonance imaging) scanning uses radio waves to build up a detailed picture of organs and tissues within the body. It uses powerful magnets to give a high resolution image allowing doctors to see clearly any areas of disease. It is also often used to check how effective previous medical treatment has been. Since the 1980s this has become an increasingly useful tool for doctors investigating the workings of the human body. A group of doctors surveyed in the USA in 2010 said MRI scans were the most useful weapon in their armoury in fighting disease.

PET scans and CT Scans

Positron emission tomography (PET) injects a slightly radioactive tracer into the bloodstream, allowing 3D colour images of tissues and bones to be seen, and is often used to investigate cancers and heart problems. Computed tomography (CT) uses many X-ray images taken at slightly different angles to produce a cross-sectional image of the area of the body, which can be used to diagnose illness or to find the location of, for example, cancerous cells. These procedures are expensive, often costing £1000 a time, and are usually used after the other scanning techniques have raised issues or complications.

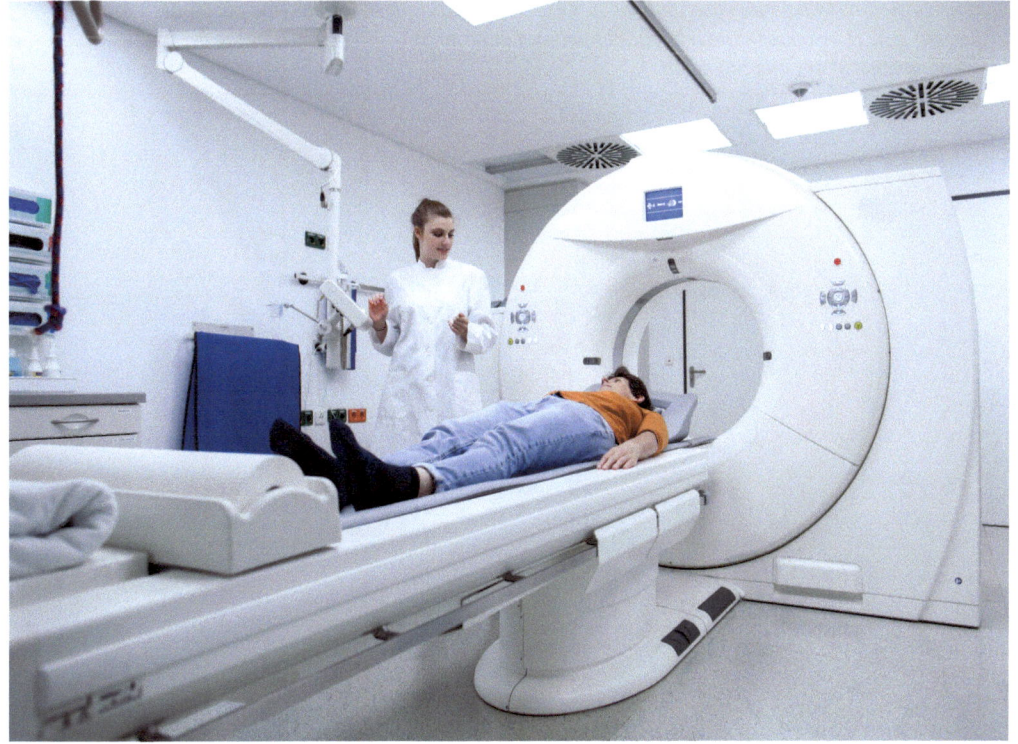

▲ **Source G:** A doctor with a patient at an MRI scanner, 2015

> **THINK**
> 1. How have these developments in scanning techniques contributed to the advance of medical knowledge over the twentieth century?
> 2. Which *one* development would you say has been most significant? Why?

The discovery of DNA and genetic research in the later twentieth century

FOCUS TASK

Complete the card as you work through the section.

Breakthrough: DNA	To what extent [1–5]
....	....
....	....

In 1953 Crick, Watson and Franklin published a paper about DNA (deoxyribonucleic acid) which carries genetic information about hereditary materials in human beings. Nearly every cell contains identical information. It is how humans reproduce themselves. In 1990 the Human Genome Project set out to build up a complete genetic blueprint of human beings; a task completed in 2003. Understanding DNA has huge implications for medical research and medical knowledge. In 1996 by copying cells (cloning) researchers were able to clone Dolly the sheep in an attempt to 'grow' medicines for humans in sheep's milk. By modifying DNA it has become possible to eliminate genetic diseases. Already genetic engineering has reversed mutations that cause blindness, stopped cancer cells from multiplying and made some cells impervious to AIDS. DNA can be used to screen people for inherited diseases, and ensure babies are born without life-threatening diseases (see Source H and Figure 4.1). Surely now scientists know most of what there is to know about disease. That must be an advance in medical knowledge.

THINK

1. What are the arguments in favour of three-parent babies?
2. What are the arguments against three-parent babies?
3. What does the issue tell us about the development of medical knowledge?

Source H: An article from *Discover Magazine*, February 2015

On Tuesday, the UK's House of Commons voted 382 to 128 in favour of the controversial technique, called mitochondrial donation, and the first 'three-person baby' could be conceived later this year. Doctors say mitochondrial donation will prevent mothers from transferring incurable genetic diseases to their children. Opponents have raised ethical concerns, saying it sets humanity on the slippery slope toward 'designer babies'. Church groups in the UK lobbied for parliament to oppose the new law. They oppose the destruction of human embryos, and worry that the law opens a Pandora's box of genetic tinkering.

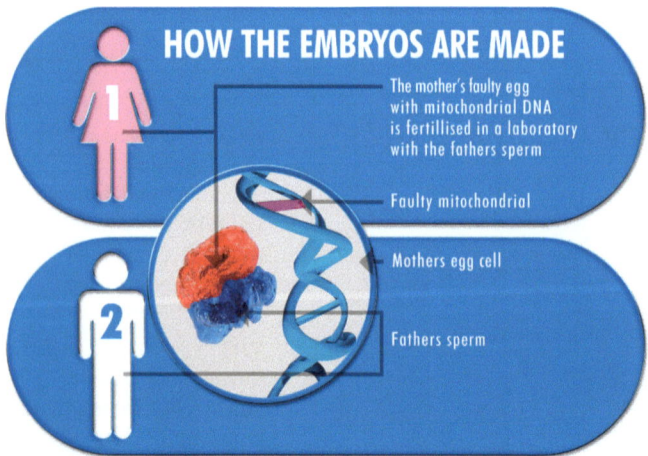
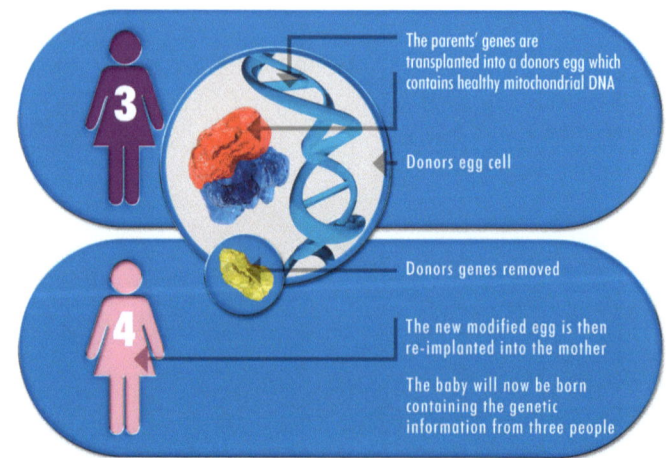

▲ Figure 4.1: How three-parent babies are made

4 Advances in medical knowledge

FOCUS TASK REVISITED

1. The focus task asked you to complete various cards to help you decide what progress has been made in medical knowledge.
2. Collect all your focus task cards and plot the information onto your personal copy of this graph:

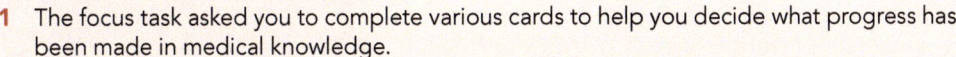

Y-axis: Massive change / Little change
X-axis: Medieval | C16th and C17th | C19th | C20th

3. Now decide which period had, in your opinion, the *most* progress in medical knowledge, and why.
4. In groups, discuss your answer to Question 3 – do you all agree or are some answers different? (How do you define 'medical progress'?)

ACTIVITY

Use your focus task cards to hold a balloon debate. Take it in turns to present the argument for each bit of medical progress on the focus task cards. At the end of each round take a vote to decide which of the bits of medical progress will be ejected from the balloon. Keep going until you have the 'best' bit of medical progress remaining.

TOPIC SUMMARY

- Medieval people did have some medical knowledge.
- Alchemists and scientists tried hard to find the 'Elixir of Life' but failed, although they did much to improve scientific techniques.
- The Renaissance was when people started to question the 'wisdom' of the Ancient World.
- People like Vesalius, Paré and Harvey radically changed the way illness was understood.
- Germ theory fundamentally altered the way people thought of disease.
- In the twentieth century techniques to 'see' inside the body revolutionised the way doctors identify illness.
- Throughout the twentieth and twenty-first centuries scientists have discovered more and more how the human body works.
- DNA and genetic engineering have introduced further advances in our understanding of illness.
- Some people think we now have too much medical knowledge.

Practice questions

1. Describe developments in medical knowledge in medieval times. *(For guidance, see page 125.)*
2. Explain why the work of Vesalius, Paré and Harvey was important in advancing medical knowledge in the sixteenth and seventeenth centuries. *(For guidance, see page 126.)*
3. Which of Sources E and F is the more useful to a historian studying developments in scanning technology over the twentieth century? *(For guidance, see page 123.)*
4. Outline how medical knowledge has changed from c.500 to the present day. *(For guidance, see page 127.)*

5 Developments in patient care

This chapter focuses on the key question: How has the care of patients improved over time?

In the UK today if you are sick and in need of medical treatment you either visit your local doctor or, for more serious illnesses, injuries or for an operation, you visit a hospital. All these services are provided under a state-run National Health Service (NHS). However, this has not always been the case. The development of these care facilities has been a very long process. During the medieval period the church dominated provision but from the mid-sixteenth century onwards voluntary and charity institutions began to take an the responsibility for nursing and patient care. During the twentieth century the government began to take an active role in looking after the welfare of its citizens and since 1948 the NHS has been in operation, treating people 'from the cradle to the grave'.

FOCUS TASK

As you work through this chapter gather together information to enable you to complete this time chart. In each section make bullet points to spell out the key features of hospitals, nursing and patient care during that period. At the end of the chapter you will be able to use this information to make a judgement upon the degree of change in patient care that has taken place.

Time period	Types of hospital available	Responsibility for running the hospital	Standard of nursing and patient care
Medieval period			
Sixteenth and seventeenth centuries			
Eighteenth century			
Nineteenth century			
Twentieth and twenty-first centuries			

The role of the church and monasteries from the medieval period up to the mid-sixteenth century

During the medieval period hospitals were essentially religious institutions whose role and functions were very different from what we expect from modern hospitals today. The principal concern of medieval hospitals was the health of the soul over the health of the body. As we have already seen, the emphasis was on care and religion rather than treatment and cure.

Almost all medieval hospitals were run by the church and the building of the monasteries during the twelfth century onwards led to an explosion in the number of hospitals set up between the twelfth and fourteenth centuries. Most monasteries included an infirmary in its layout, such as that of Tintern Abbey on the Welsh border (see Figure 5.1). Throughout England and Wales over 1100 hospitals were set up during the medieval period. These hospitals varied greatly in size – many were small, containing no more than a dozen patients, while a few were larger, such as St Leonard's in York which, by 1287, could accommodate 225 sick patients.

5 Developments in patient care

> **THINK**
> Study the plan of Tintern Abbey (Figure 5.1) What evidence can you find to prove that monasteries played an important role in the care of sick people during the medieval period?

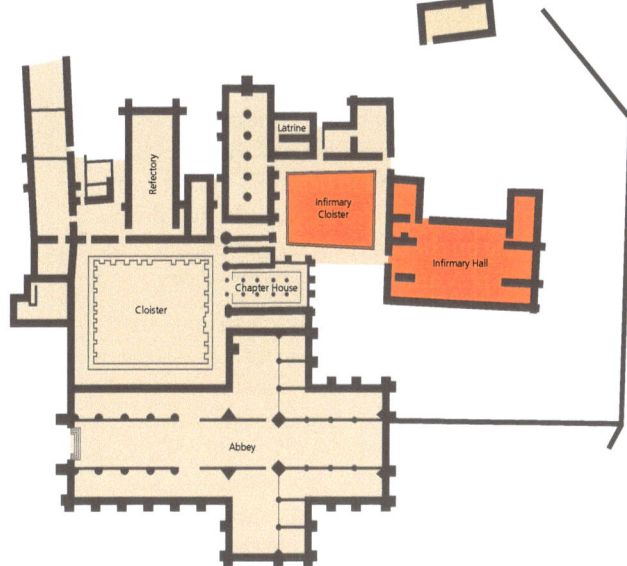

Figure 5.1: A plan of Tintern Abbey which was constructed in stages between the late twelfth and late thirteenth century. The infirmary (red) was an important part of the monastery

Different types of hospitals in medieval times

The medieval period witnessed a growth in hospitals but only about 10 per cent of them actually cared for sick people (see Figure 5.2). They were called hospitals because they provided 'hospitality', a place of rest and recuperation but not a place to be cured. Some specialised in looking after certain types of people, such as lepers, while others such as St Bartholomew's in London looked after destitute women who were pregnant and supported the infants of mothers who had died during childbirth.

Leper hospitals

A common incurable and contagious disease during the medieval period was leprosy and a great leprosy epidemic during the twelfth and thirteenth centuries brought about a growth of specific leprosy hospitals. Leprosy inflicted horrible deformities on its victims and they were forced to wear special clothes and ring a warning bell as they walked, and they were not allowed to marry. Many people feared lepers and thought that those with the disease were being punished by God. Leper hospitals were built on the outskirts of towns to limit the mixing with the rest of the population. They provided lodging and food but no treatment.

> **Source A:** A local law enforced in the town of Berwick-upon-Tweed in an attempt to stop the spread of leprosy
>
> *No leper shall come within the gates of the borough and if one gets in by chance, the serjeant shall put him out at once. If one wilfully forces his way in, his clothes shall be taken off him and burnt and he shall be turned out naked.*

Almshouses

Almshouses were the medieval equivalent of the modern care home and they were a response to an aging population. Almshouses offered sheltered accommodation and basic nursing, but no medical treatment.

Most were very small, sometimes just a priest and up to a dozen inmates. Most occupants were older needing long-term care, but they also contained widows with young children or single pregnant women. Almshouses also gave shelter to travellers and the poor, who would be given a few nights accommodation.

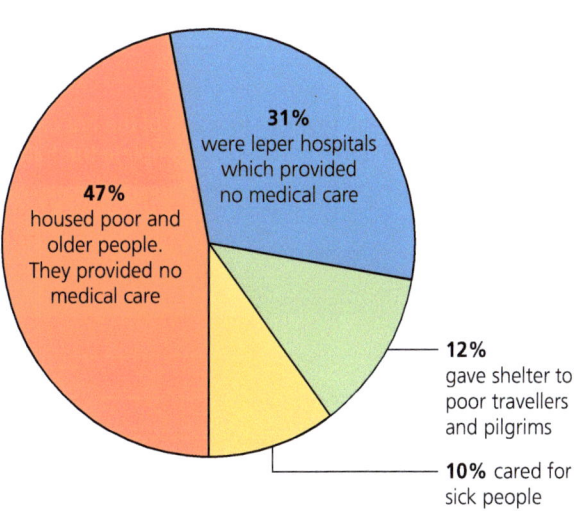

Figure 5.2: Pie-chart showing the type of patient care provided during the medieval period

65

Christian hospitals

Christian hospitals were set up, paid for and run by the church and they looked after poor people as well as sick people. They did not treat sickness but aimed to make the patients as comfortable as they could. People who were seriously ill and in need of constant care were often not allowed in as they would stop people concentrating on the main purpose of the hospital which was to pray and attend religious services.

Hospitals provided basic nursing, clean and quiet conditions, regular meals and warmth, and sometimes surgery and medicine. The staff were brothers and sisters in religious orders. They cared for sick people and tried to save their souls, but they did not attempt to cure them. There were few, if any, doctors. The staff at St Leonard's in York consisted of several chaplains but no doctors. St Bartholomew's, which had been founded in London in 1123, did not appoint its first doctor until the sixteenth century.

Hospitals were religious institutions and were often referred to as 'Houses of God'. When Walter Suffield, the Bishop of Norwich, left money in his will of 1257 for the construction of the 'Great Hospital' he did so because he believed it was his Christian duty to help sick, homeless and poor people (see Figure 5.3). He also wanted to cleanse himself of his sins to ensure he entered heaven when he died.

Patients were expected to spend much of their day praying and confessing their sins. It was believed that they were poor and sick because they had sinned and they now needed to rid themselves of their sins. This was the function of the hospital. If they prayed, showed that they repented their sins and said prayers for the people who had donated money to the hospital, they would be helped into heaven after death.

The hospital consisted of a hall full of beds, at the end of which were small chapels where monks said mass. Nuns and helpers attended the patients.

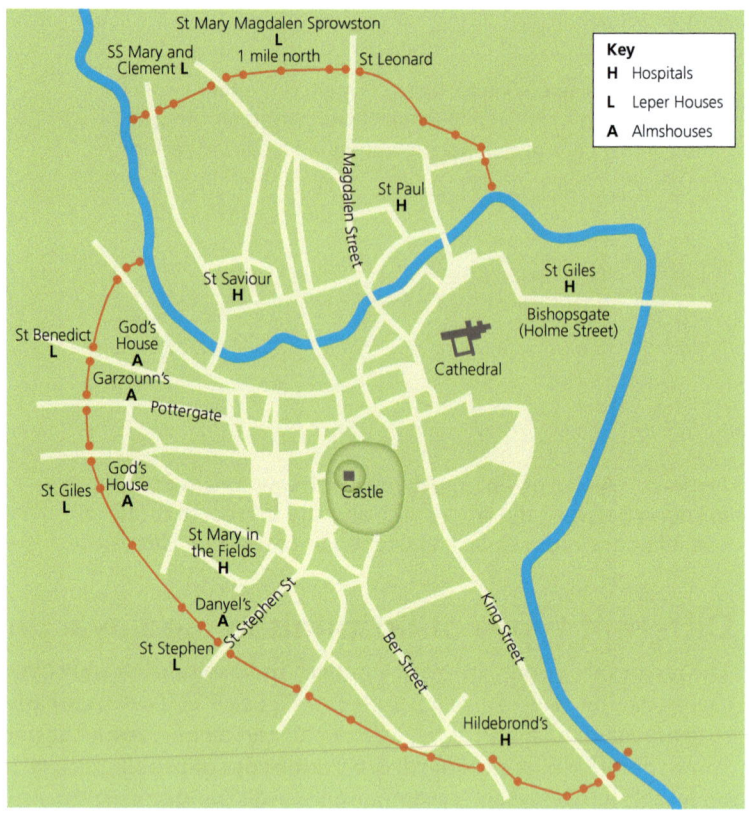

▲ Figure 5.3: A map of medieval Norwich showing leper houses, almshouses and hospitals

Source B: An extract from the rules of the hospital of St John in Bridgwater, Somerset, in 1219

No lepers, lunatics, or persons having the falling sickness or other contagious disease, and no pregnant women, or sucking infants, and no intolerable persons, even though they be poor and infirm, are to be admitted in the hospital; and if any such be admitted by mistake, they are to be expelled as soon as possible. And when the other poor and infirm persons have recovered they are to be let out without delay.

THINK

1. Use the information in this section to think about the role and function of the hospital during the medieval period, making use of the information in Sources A (page 65) and B and Figure 5.3 to complete the following table.

	What does this source tell you about the types of medical care on offer during the medieval period?	What does this source tell us about the role and function of this type of hospital?	What does this source tell us about attitudes towards the care of sick people?
Source A			
Source B			
Figure 5.3			

2. 'The Christian church was concerned with the care rather than the cure of sick people.' How far do you agree with this statement?

The roles of voluntary charities in patient care after the mid-sixteenth century

The mid-sixteenth century onwards witnessed a decline in the role of the church in administering patient care and the growth of voluntary charities taking on that role, especially after the closure of the monasteries.

The impact of the closure of the monasteries

When Henry VIII ordered the dissolution of the monasteries in the 1530s it resulted in the closure of many hospitals and this had a dramatic impact upon patient care. The church now ceased to be a supporter of hospitals and that role now had to be taken on by voluntary charities.

In some areas town or city councils stepped in to take over the running of almshouses that looked after older poor people and the hospital, which took care of the poor in general. In London the authorities petitioned the crown to provide funds to endow hospitals such as St Bartholomew's, St Thomas' and St Mary's to enable them to continue to provide services of patient care for their communities. In providing royal funds, it proved to be the first occasion when secular support was provided for medical institutions.

The creation of 'royal hospitals' in London

Across London a total of five major hospitals were endowed with royal funds during the mid-sixteenth century to enable them to continue to administer care for sick and poor people of the capital. The endowment usually took the form of the granting of land, which could then be rented out to provide the institution with a steady, though often insufficient, income.

St Bartholomew's Hospital

The dissolution of the monasteries left St Barts in a difficult position as it took away its income. In a bid to keep the hospital open, the city authorities petitioned the king and in December 1546 the institution was granted to the Corporation of the City of London by royal charter of Henry VIII and endowed with properties, land and other income entitlements. The hospital served the poor of the area of West Smithfield.

St Mary Bethlehem (including Bethlem)

St Mary Bethlehem, which included Bethlem Hospital, was dissolved in the late 1530s. In 1546 the Lord Mayor of London, Sir John Gresham, petitioned the crown to grant both institutions to the city. A royal charter was granted in 1547. The Bethlem site concentrated upon looking after the mentally insane.

St Thomas' Hospital

St Thomas' hospital, which had originally been founded c.1100 by a mixed order of Augustinian monks and nuns, provided shelter and treatment for the poor, sick and homeless in the area of Southwark. The monastery was dissolved in 1539 and its hospital closed. With nothing to take its place, the city of London authorities petitioned the crown and in 1551 King Edward VI granted the site by royal charter and the hospital re-opened that year. It quickly re-established itself as a hospital for poor people who were ill, but also took on the responsibility for treating patients suffering from venereal disease.

Christ's Hospital

Christ's Hospital was founded in 1553 by Edward VI, in the old Grey Friars' buildings in Newgate, London, in response to calls from the bishop of London to provide for the poor. It offered shelter, clothing and food to fatherless children, alongside rudimentary education.

Bridewell hospital

The fifth 'royal hospital' was that of Bridewell hospital and prison. Located on the banks of the Fleet river, it received its royal charter in 1553 and had two purposes, the housing of homeless children and the punishment of the disorderly poor.

Endowed voluntary hospitals outside London

The creation of voluntary hospitals did not just take place in London. In towns across the country it was left to the local councils to organise endowments to keep their hospitals open. In Norwich, for example, when Henry VIII ordered the closure of the monastery of St Giles and, with it, its hospital, the town council petitioned the crown.

The hospital was re-founded by a royal charter granted in 1547, which handed control of the hospital to the town corporation. The charter stated that four women were to be employed to 'make the beddes, washe and attend upon the seid poore persons'. During the following century the hospital was transformed from a religious institution into a hospital which, for the first time in its history, began to employ medical staff. By the 1570s the medical staff consisted of a barber (who let blood), a surgeon and a bonesetter. Medical care was now being focused upon its patients.

> **THINK**
> 1. How did the responsibility of care for sick and poor people change after the dissolution of the monasteries in the 1530s?
> 2. 'Hospitals in London during the late sixteenth century began to specialise in the care of particular types of patients.' What evidence can you find to support this statement?

Science and the development of endowed hospitals in the eighteenth century

During the eighteenth century new hospitals were opened, paid for by private individuals, charities or town councils. A number of factors influenced the growth in the provision of hospital care during this century.

The development of scientific enquiry

This period witnessed a growth in scientific enquiry which in turn resulted in a growing interest in medical issues. The founding of the Royal Society in London in 1662 and various medical societies, such as the one established in Edinburgh in 1732, did much to encourage new scientific discoveries. These new societies provided opportunities to discuss ideas about medicine and to analyse and evaluate the results of experiments or trials in new surgical processes. The desire to investigate, experiment and report led to the growth of the Enlightenment, an age of scientific advancement and enquiry, a period which saw the advancement in medical knowledge.

The impact of the Industrial Revolution

Industrial development resulted in several consequences, one of which was a sharp rise in population levels. As the new industrial towns expanded so there was a corresponding demand for increased hospital provision. Part of that demand was met through financial donations from new wealthy industrialists. They wished to use their new wealth to fund the establishment of hospitals, believing that God had given them the responsibility to improve the lives of the poor and sick. One of these early philanthropists was Thomas Guy, a wealthy printer and bookseller who financed the establishment of Guy's Hospital in 1724. He held the Christian belief that the rich should help the poor, and through receiving such help, the poor would be provided with the opportunity to live cleaner and more disciplined lives.

The setting up of endowed hospitals

During the first half of the eighteenth century many new voluntary hospitals were opened, paid for by private individuals like Guy, local charities or town councils who provided the new institutions with endowments to fund their upkeep. Eleven new hospitals were founded in London during this period and a further 46 across the country in the growing industrial towns and cities (see Table 5.1).

Date	Hospital	Location	Endowed by
1719	Westminster Hospital	London	Funded by a private bank, C. Hoare & Co
1724	Guy's Hospital	London	Bequest of a wealthy businessman, Thomas Guy
1729	Royal Infirmary Hospital	Edinburgh	Wealthy patrons of Edinburgh donated funds
1735	Royal Infirmary Hospital	Bristol	Funded by Paul Fisher, a wealthy city merchant
1739	The Foundling Hospital	Bloomsbury, London	Founded by Thomas Coram, a sea captain. He wished the hospital to look after deserted young children
1752	Royal Infirmary Hospital	Manchester	Funded by Charles White, a physician, and Joseph Bancroft, a wealthy industrialist
1766	Addenbrooke's Hospital	Cambridge	Dr John Addenbrooke left £4500 in his will to set up a hospital
1779	The General Hospital	Birmingham	Donations from wealthy landowners and industrialists, including Matthew Boulton

▲ Table 5.1: Examples of some of the endowed hospitals set up during the eighteenth century

5 Developments in patient care

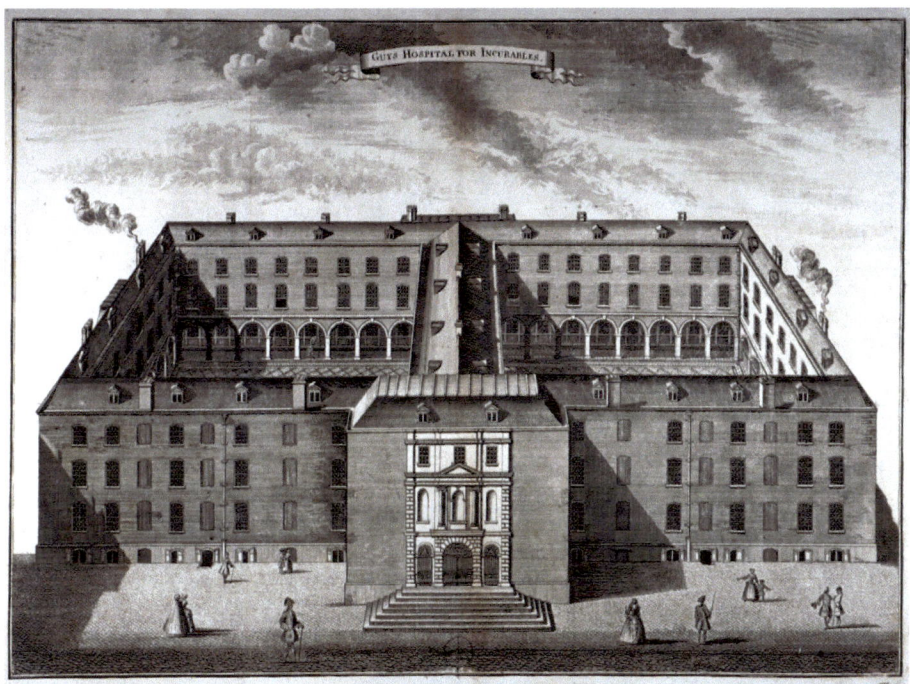

◀ **Source C:** An engraving from the 1820s showing Guy's Hospital in London. This was one of the first voluntary endowed hospitals to be established in 1724

> **Source D:** The rules of Guy's Hospital, issued after its foundation in 1724
>
> *The sick must acknowledge the goodness of God in providing so comfortable a situation, care, medicine and skill, while under the afflicting hand of God. They must behave soberly and religiously as Christians.*

The role and function of endowed hospitals

The establishment of endowed hospitals marked a turning point in the development of the hospital. They now evolved from a place to provide basic care of sick people to a centre in which to treat illness and conditions that required surgery. Some of them became centres for the education and training of doctors and surgeons.

Within these institutions the primary role was to look after the poor sick, as people with money normally paid for a doctor and nurse to treat them privately at home. The patients were looked after by nursing helpers who undertook the manual work and ensured that the patients were washed, kept warm and fed regularly. Nursing sisters were able to treat ill patients with herbal remedies. Simple surgery such as the removal of bladder stones and the setting of broken bones was carried out by physicians. Treatment was normally free.

Another function of the hospital was the issue of medicines. During the 1770s a number of dispensaries were set up – the Public Dispensary of Edinburgh in 1776, the Metropolitan Dispensary and Charitable Fund in 1779 and the Finsbury Dispensary in 1780, both in central London.

> **THINK**
>
> 1. What do Sources C and D tell us about hospitals in the eighteenth century?
> 2. The growth in the provision of hospital care during the eighteenth century was influenced by developments such as:
>   - scientific enquiry
>   - industrial development
>   - funding by private individuals.
>
>   Arrange these developments in order of their significance in influencing the growth in hospital provision. Explain your choices.

Changes in the nineteenth century

Two important developments in patient care occurred during the nineteenth century. One was the emergence of nursing as a profession and the other was the planned design of hospitals. Both of these developments were heavily influenced by one individual – Florence Nightingale.

Growth in the number of hospitals

As the country's population continued to grow throughout the nineteenth century the pressure to provide medical care resulted in the establishment of general hospitals in cities across the country. In 1800 there were approximately 3000 patients in hospitals across England and Wales and by 1851 this figure had risen to 7619. Specialist hospitals had also begun to appear, dealing with such areas as maternity care, orthopaedics, and eyes, nose and throat (see Table 5.2). By the 1860s the cottage hospital movement had resulted in the setting up of small hospitals in rural areas run by general practitioners.

Date of foundation	Developments in specific medical care
1800	Royal College of Surgeons opened
1814	London Chest Hospital
1828	Royal 'Free' Hospital founded by William Marsden
1834	Westminster Medical School
1851	Royal 'Marsden' Cancer Hospital
1852	Great Ormond Street Children's Hospital
1860	Nightingale School of Nursing

▲ Table 5.2: Major hospitals and specialist training institutions established between 1800 and 1900

Conditions within these new hospitals

While there was a growth in the number of hospitals, conditions for the patients within them were generally poor. Cramped, stuffy wards helped infections to spread quickly, and the fact that the wards were seldom cleaned meant that the death rate from infection was high. The quality of nursing was poor, with untrained nurses securing reputations for being dirty, ignorant and often drunk. They received little, if any, training and were often ignorant of the most basic standards of hygiene. The most common complaints waged against nurses were that they were too often dirty and drunk (see Source E). Many thought nursing was a job only for uneducated women who could do nothing else. Nursing was not looked upon as a respected profession and was certainly not seen as a career for a respectable young woman like Florence Nightingale.

> **Source E:** A description of nursing at St Bartholomew's hospital in London in 1877. It was written in 1902 by a nurse who had been a sister in the hospital in the 1870s
>
> *Drunkenness was very common among the staff nurses, who chiefly were of charwoman type, frequently of bad character, with little education. Nursing, as you understand it now, was unknown. Patients were not nursed, they were attended to, more or less. The work was hard – lockers and tables to scrub every day. We did not scrub the floors. The patients had their beds made once a day, and you thought nothing of changing fourteen or fifteen* **poultices** *two or three times a day. The nurses never used a thermometer, the dressers and clerks took the temperatures.*

> **THINK**
>
> 'The first half of the nineteenth century saw the opening of many new hospitals but these hospitals did not bring about any improvement in patient care.' What evidence can you find in this section to support this statement?

Florence Nightingale and the professionalisation of nursing

As we have seen, during the first half of the nineteenth century standards of nursing were very poor. What changed nursing were the actions of a number of females – Florence Nightingale, Mary Seacole and Betsi Cadwaladr – all of whom took part in the nursing of British soldiers during the Crimean War (1854–6).

The impact of the Crimean War

The Crimean War was the first war in which reporters sent back reports to newspapers in Britain using the new telegraph system and the public soon began reading about the awful conditions experienced by sick and wounded British soldiers fighting in the Crimea. What got Florence Nightingale interested in the war were the reports she read in *The Times*.

Born into a wealthy family, Nightingale believed God had wanted her to be a nurse and despite opposition from her parents she had trained as a nurse in Germany and in Paris during the early 1850s. After returning to England she worked in several hospitals before the outbreak of the Crimean War in 1854.

> **Source F:** Shortly after her arrival in Scutari, Florence Nightingale wrote to Sydney Herbert, describing the conditions in which wounded and sick soldiers were treated. Her letter is dated 25 November 1854
>
> *It appears that in these hospitals the washing of linen and of the men are considered a minor detail. No washing has been performed for the men or the bed – except by ourselves. When we came here, there was neither basin, towel, nor soap in the Wards. The consequences of this are Fever, Cholera, Gangrene, Lice, Bugs, Fleas.*

Florence Nightingale goes to the Crimea

Having secured government funding, Nightingale took 38 of the best nurses she could find and travelled to the British military hospital at Scutari on the Black Sea coast of Turkey. Upon their arrival at Scutari on 4 November 1854 they were appalled by what they saw. There were 1700 wounded and sick soldiers in the field hospital, many of whom were suffering from cholera and typhoid, housed in filthy wards. There were not enough beds or medical supplies. Added to this problem was the fact that the army doctors resented Nightingale's presence and opposed her interference.

However, Nightingale had the support of both Sydney Herbert, Minister of War Supplies, and Dr Andrew Smith, head of the Army Medical Department. Dr Smith ensured that she obtained sufficient supplies of the medical items she needed, and she also had financial backing from *The Times*, which reported upon her improvements.

One of Nightingale's first tasks was to clean the wards. Patients were given a regular wash, clean clothes and had their bedding changed regularly. To help prevent the spread of disease, patients were separated according to their illness, plenty of space was put between each bed and fresh air circulated from open windows. These measures had dramatic results. After just six months only 100 of the 1700 patients were still confined to bed, and the death rate in the hospital had fallen from 42 in every 100 patients to 2 in every 100. Through these reforms Nightingale had laid down new standards of patient care.

> **THINK**
> 1. What do Sources F and G tell you about conditions for sick and wounded soldiers in army hospitals at the start of the Crimean War in 1854?
> 2. Describe the changes made by Florence Nightingale to the care of sick and wounded soldiers in the army hospital at Scutari.

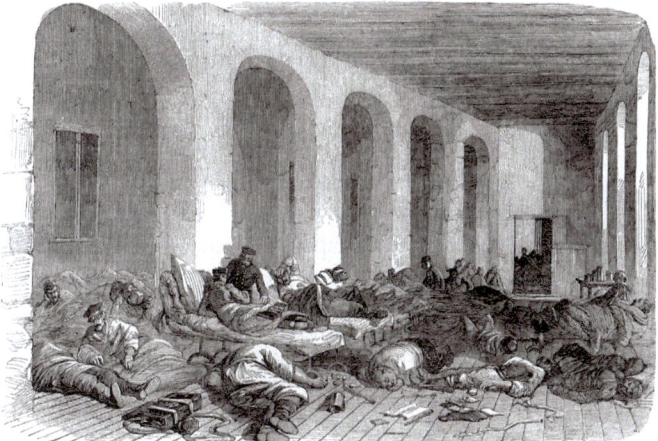

▲ **Source G:** Conditions in the military hospital at Scutari in 1854 before the arrival of Florence Nightingale

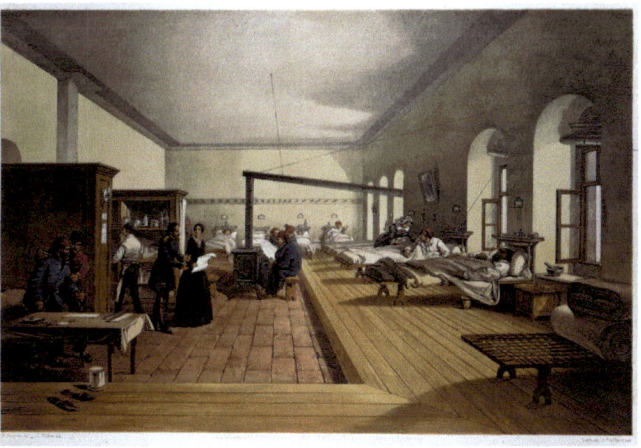

▲ **Source H:** A hospital ward at Scutari in 1856 showing the changes to patient care introduced by Florence Nightingale

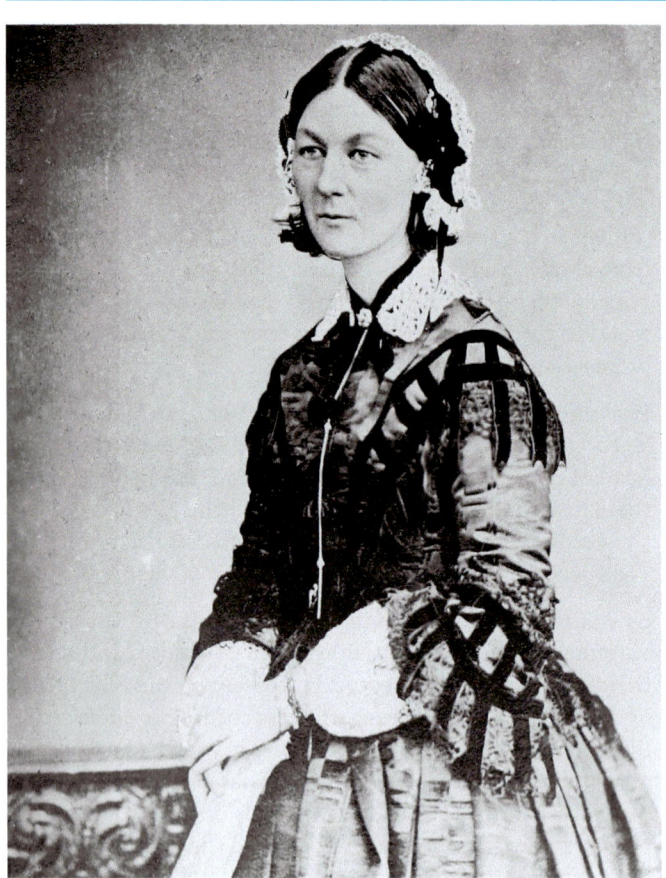

▲ Source 1: Florence Nightingale

Florence Nightingale and the birth of modern nursing

Upon her return to Britain in 1856 Nightingale set up a public fund and was successful in raising nearly £50,000. Much of this was used to set up the Nightingale School of Nursing in a wing of St Thomas' Hospital in London.

In 1859 she published *Notes on Nursing*, which set out the training nurses should receive. The training was very practical and ward based. Training in the school was very strict:

- Nurses were only allowed to go out in pairs.
- They had to live in at the hospital.
- They had to keep a diary of their work, which was inspected every month.

They were taught to be as clean as possible, to change dressings and to be proper assistants to doctors and surgeons. Instead of being minders and cleaners as they had been in the past, nurses were now to be seen as an essential part of patient care and treatment. By 1900 nursing schools had opened around the country using Nightingale's ideas.

Florence Nightingale influences the design of new hospitals

In 1863 Nightingale published *Notes on Hospitals*, which introduced new ideas about the design of hospitals. She believed that new hospitals should consider the importance of 'the proper use of fresh air, light, warmth, cleanliness, quiet and the proper selection and administration of diets'. When St Thomas' Hospital was rebuilt in 1868 it became one of the first hospitals to adopt the 'pavilion principle' devised by Nightingale. This consisted of six separate wards at right angles to a long, linked corridor which encouraged good circulation of air.

The importance of Florence Nightingale

In 1850 there had been no trained nurses in Britain, yet by 1901 there were 68,000. In 1899 the International Council of Nurses was set up in London. Nursing had finally been recognised as a profession, in large part due to the efforts of Florence Nightingale. Hospital design had also undergone radical change. By the end of the nineteenth century many towns and cities had built new hospitals and in their design they embodied many of the recommendations put forward by Florence Nightingale.

THINK

1. Explain **two** changes introduced by Florence Nightingale which improved the quality of nursing.
2. What key features did Florence Nightingale consider to be essential in the design of new hospitals? Explain why.

Problems in 1850	Solutions found by 1900
Untrained nurses	Trained nurses
Lack of respect for nurses	Nursing recognised as a profession
Cramped, stuffy wards	Spacious, light and well-ventilated wards
Poor sanitation, toilet facilities and sewage disposal	Good sanitation, connected to main drains and piped water supplies
Lack of cleanliness	Clean wards
Unhygienic surgery and dressings	Aseptic surgery and dressings

▲ Table 5.3: Changes in nursing and hospitals between 1850 and 1900

5 Developments in patient care

The contribution of Mary Seacole (1805–81)

Another nurse who made her mark in the Crimean War was Mary Seacole. The daughter of a Scottish sailor, Seacole was born in Kingston, Jamaica, where her mother ran a medical centre for British soldiers and sailors on the island, and Seacole soon developed a keen interest in nursing. She travelled to Britain in 1854 and volunteered her services to the army in the Crimea.

In 1855 she opened the 'British Hospital' between Balaclava and Sebastopol to treat wounded and sick soldiers. She dealt with jaundice, diarrhoea, dysentery and frostbite, and was often seen going into the thick of the battle with her medicine bag. When the war ended she returned to Britain and in 1857 published an autobiography, *The Wonderful Adventures of Mrs Seacole in Many Lands*, which helped to raise awareness of the contribution of nursing during the Crimean War.

The contribution of Betsi Cadwaladr (1789–1860)

Like Seacole, Betsi Cadwaladr helped with the nursing of soldiers in the Crimea. Born in Bala in north Wales in 1789, Cadwaladr was one of 16 children. At the age of 14 she ran away from home, travelled to Liverpool and then to London where she became interested in nursing. Between 1815 and 1820 she served as a maid to a ship's captain, which enabled her to travel to South America, Africa and Australia. Upon her return to London she trained as a nurse and in 1854, aged 65, she went to the Crimea to help nurse the wounded soldiers. She did not get on well with Florence Nightingale and so moved from the hospital at Scutari to Balaclava. She cleaned wounds and changed bandages, working from 6 a.m. to 11 p.m. However, the war took its toll on her health and she caught cholera and dysentery. She had to leave the Crimea in 1855 and died in 1860. The Betsi Cadwaladr NHS Trust in north Wales commemorates her.

> **THINK**
>
> To what extent were Mary Seacole and Betsi Cadwaladr important in the history of nursing?

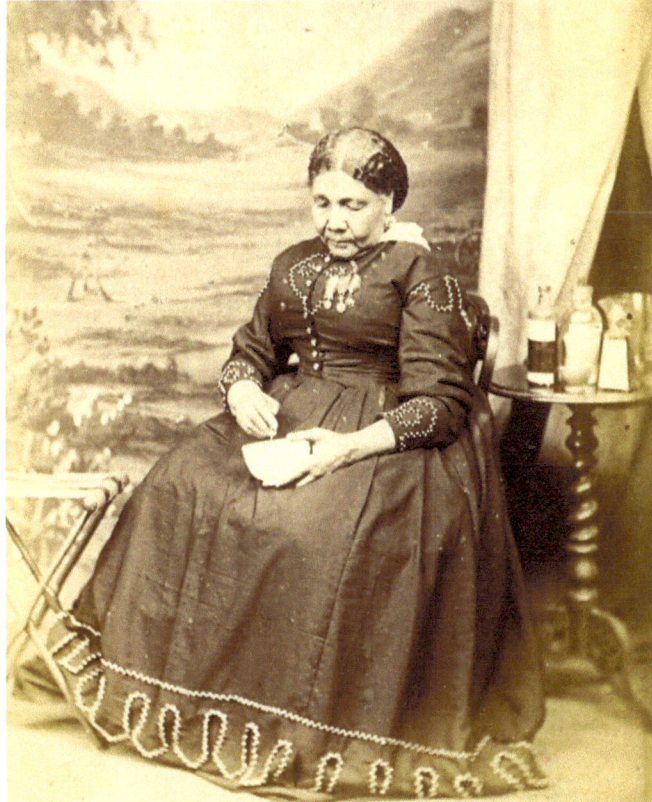

▲ **Source J:** Mary Seacole

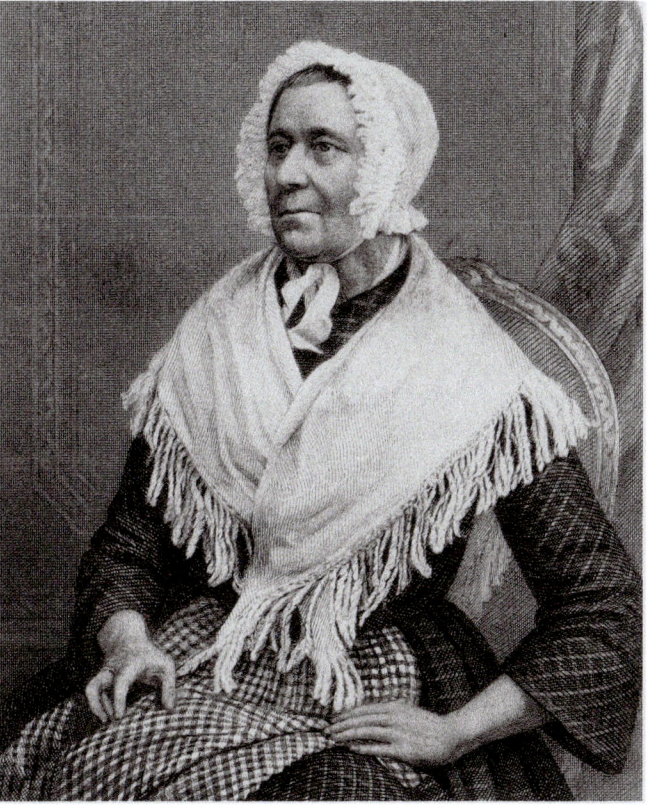

▲ **Source K:** Betsi Cadwaladr

The impact of the early twentieth century Liberal reforms

The early decades of the twentieth century witnessed the beginnings of the creation of the **Welfare State** when the government began to take some responsibility for managing the care and treatment of sick people and those in need.

Changes in government attitude

During the nineteenth century governments had traditionally followed a policy of *laissez-faire*, believing it was not their job to interfere with people's lives unless they really had to. During the early twentieth century, however, attitudes began to change and the Liberal governments of 1906–14 broke with the past and introduced a series of welfare reforms designed to help people who fell into difficulty through sickness, old age or unemployment. The reforms tackled such areas as the provision of education, the medical inspection of school pupils, workers, compensation rights and the provision of old-age pensions (see Table 5.4).

Year	Act passed	Effect of legislation
1906	Workmen's Compensation Act	Granted compensation for injury at work
	Education (Provision of Meals) Act	Introduced free school meals
1907	Education (Administrative Provisions) Act	Created school medical inspections
	Matrimonial Causes Act	Maintenance payments to be paid to divorced women
1908	Children and Young Person's Act (Children's Charter)	Made it illegal to sell alcohol, tobacco or fireworks to children
	Old-Age Pensions Act	Over 70s received 5 shillings a week (25p), 7 shillings and 6 pence for a married couple
1909	Labour Exchanges Act	Helped get people back into a job
	Housing and Town Planning Act	Made it illegal to build back-to-back houses
1911	National Insurance Act	Sick and unemployment pay introduced if you paid contributions into the scheme

▲ Table 5.4: Early twentieth-century Liberal reforms

> **THINK**
> Study Source L.
> - What happens to children's weight in term time?
> - What happens to children's weight in holiday time?
> - Does this source suggest providing free school meals for 'necessitous children' worked?
> - Does this source prove that the Liberal welfare reforms worked?

Case study: School meals in Bradford

Manchester and Bradford local authorities had introduced school meals for 'necessitous children' and led the campaign for the introduction of school meals nationally. One of the first things the Liberal government did in 1906 was to introduce free school meals, but it was not compulsory for local authorities to provide them until 1914, when 14 million were served over the course of the year. Parents could be asked to make a contribution towards the cost if they could afford it, and the rest of the money had to come from local rates.

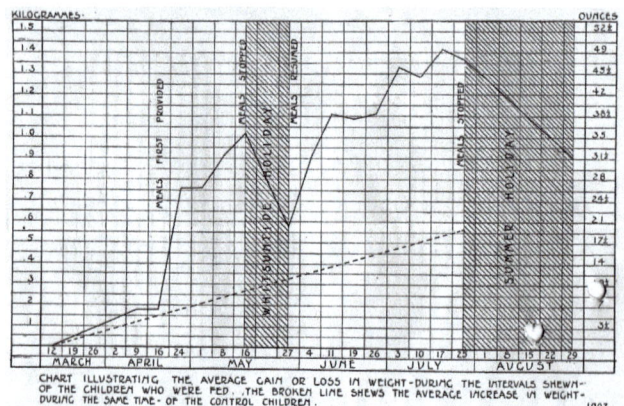

◄ Source L: Extract from a report by the City of Bradford medical officer on the effects of school meals, 1907

5 Developments in patient care

What were the achievements of the Liberal government of 1906–14?

In introducing the 1909 Budget, Lloyd George stated: 'This is a war budget ... to wage implacable warfare against poverty and squalidness.' But did these measures have as much impact as he stated they would? Medical inspections were introduced in 1907, but poor families could not afford to pay for necessary treatment. Pensions were introduced for over 70s (the average age of death was around 50), but only if you had worked all your life and could prove you were not a drunkard. The National Insurance scheme only applied if you paid regular contributions, but part of the cause of poverty was irregular employment. The 1909 Budget was thrown out in the House of Lords by the Conservative peers, who were opposed to paying for these reforms. It caused a constitutional crisis. Even some Liberals thought they were too expensive. And others, like those in the newly formed Labour Party, felt they did not go far enough.

The National Insurance Act 1911

Among the most significant was the introduction of the National Insurance Act 1911, which laid down the first steps towards the creation of a welfare state. The minister responsible for this Act was David Lloyd George, the Chancellor of the Exchequer. Lloyd George proposed an insurance scheme which involved workers and their employers making weekly contributions into a central fund which was used to give workers sickness benefit and free medical care from a panel doctor if they became ill. Those workers contributing into the scheme would be entitled to receive free medical attention and a payment of 10 shillings (50p) per week for 26 weeks if absent from work due to illness, after which a disability pension of 5 shillings (25p) paid weekly would be available. Many doctors, however, opposed the scheme but Lloyd George got over the opposition by paying each doctor more money for each patient they saw.

A second National Insurance Act was passed in 1913 which extended the scheme to include unemployment insurance. This allowed workers who became unemployed to claim unemployment benefit of 7 shillings per week up to a maximum of 15 weeks.

While this was a major step forward in providing welfare care it also had its limitations. The scheme was restricted to certain trades and occupations and it did not cover families (wives and children), only the insured husbands. Neither did it cover unemployed, older, mentally ill or chronically ill people.

Welfare care during the 1920s and 1930s

After the First World War Lloyd George, who was now Prime Minister, promised 'a land fit for heroes' and he initiated a building programme for over 200,000 new houses to be built by 1922 to replace slum housing. He also extended National Insurance to cover a greater proportion of the workforce, allowing insured persons to claim both sickness and unemployment benefit. The payments came to be known as the dole.

During the economic depression of the 1930s it became harder to get good medical care and the government even reduced its contributions to health insurance. Many unemployed people failed to keep up with their contributions into the scheme and by 1934 there were 4 million insurance policies on which people owed payments. As people had little money they were forced to rely on cheap, easy-to-obtain remedies which had been handed down through the generations.

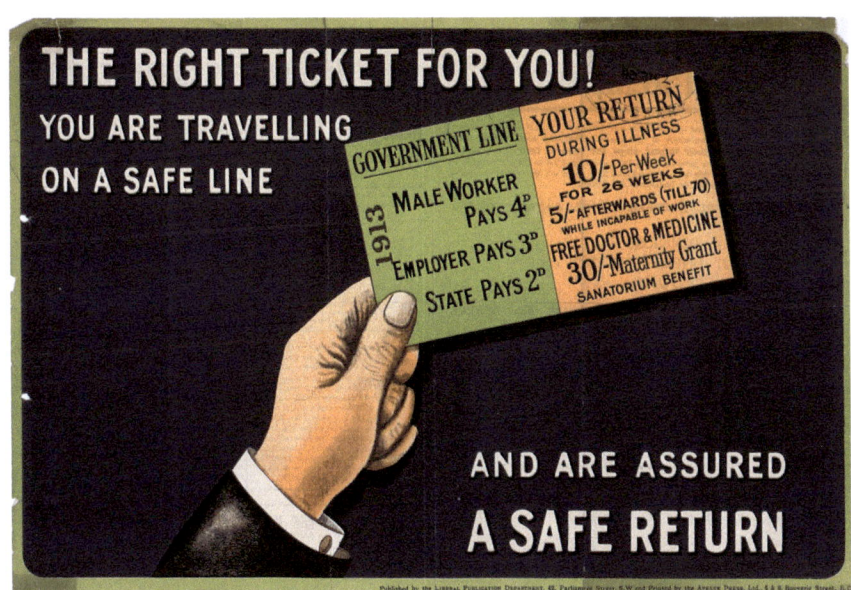

> **THINK**
>
> 1 Why were the Liberal reforms so divisive?
> 2 Which of the reforms do you think might be most successful? Why?
> 3 What can you learn from Source M about the National Insurance Act 1911?
> 4 To what extent does the National Insurance Act 1911 mark a change in government attitudes towards the welfare of its citizens?

◀ Source M: A government leaflet issued in 1911 to explain how the new National Insurance Scheme would work

The Beveridge Report

Lloyd George and the Liberal governments of 1906–14 had set up a free health service for insured workers but their wives and children had to pay for any treatment they needed. Visits to and from the doctor, medicine, spectacles and dental treatment all had to be paid for. During the Second World War questions began to be asked about how medical care should be best organised once the war was over.

The Beveridge Report, 1942

In June 1941 the wartime government set up a committee to look into welfare provision and it was chaired by William Beveridge, a man who had helped formulate the Liberal welfare reforms of 1906–14. The Beveridge Report was published in December 1942 and it became a best seller with over 600,000 copies sold. It identified 'five evil giants' that needed to be tackled by government action and these were 'Want, Disease, Ignorance, Squalor and Idleness'. While Churchill, the wartime Conservative Prime Minister, was reluctant to act upon the suggestions of the report, the Labour Party, under its leader Clement Attlee, promised to put the proposals into action if it was elected after the war.

Tackling the 'five evil giants'

When the Labour Party was elected into office after a landslide victory in July 1945 it immediately set about implementing the recommendations of the Beveridge Report. It passed a number of Acts which together helped establish the 'Welfare State'.

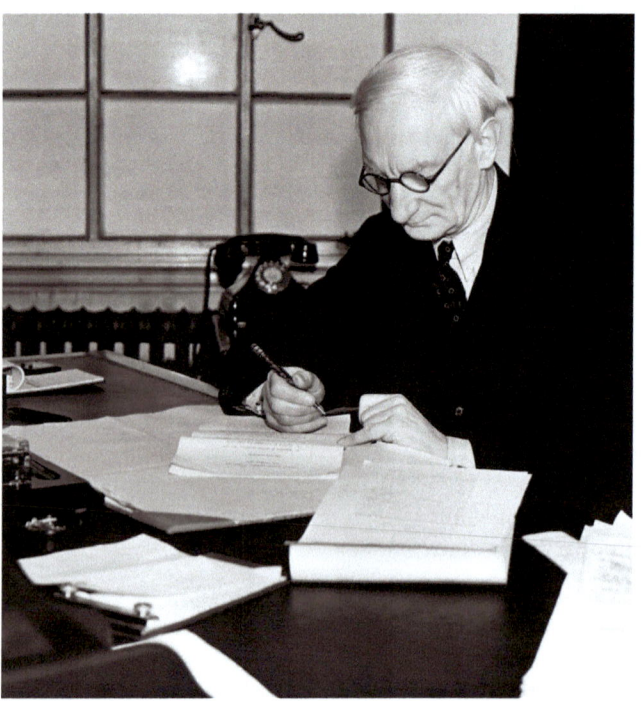

▲ **Source N:** William Beveridge, in 1942, economist and social reformer

Battle against want
- National Insurance Act 1946 provided benefits for unemployed people and pregnant women, pensions for retired people, allowances for sick people, those who had been widowed, and mothers and children

Battle against squalor
- 1946 and 1949 Housing Acts provided financial aid to local authorities to rebuild towns and cities and provided for the building of council houses
- 1946 New Towns Act allowed for the construction of 14 new towns
- 1949 Access to the Countryside Act

Battle against idleness and ignorance
- 1944 Education Act provided free primary and secondary education
- 1947 School leaving age raised to 15 in 1947
- 1948 Employment and Training Act attempted to establish a skilled workforce

Battle against disease
- 1946 National Health Service Act proposed the setting up of a free health service for all

> **THINK**
>
> How did the Labour government of 1945–51 deal with the 'five evil giants' identified by Beveridge?

Provision under the NHS after 1946

The National Health Service Act 1946 is considered to be the foundation stone in the creation of the Welfare State. The aim of the Act was to set up a health service that was to be 'free of charge' and available to everyone. The main features of the Act were:

- for the first time every British citizen could have free medical treatment – hospitals, doctors, nurses, pharmacists, opticians and dentists were brought together under one umbrella organisation
- all hospitals were to be brought under state control (nationalisation) under the control of the Ministry of Health
- consultants in hospitals received salaries and all treatment to patients in hospitals was to be free
- a national system of general practitioners (GPs) was to be set up and they, along with dentists and opticians, were to receive fees according to the numbers of patients on their registers, not according to the treatment given. All treatment was to be free to the patient
- health centres were to be set up – local authorities were paid to provide vaccinations, maternity care, district nurses, health visitors and ambulances
- the aim was to provide support 'from the cradle to the grave', financed out of taxation through the payment of National Insurance contributions.

These changes, announced in 1946, took two years to complete. A major reason for this was because the Minster for Health, Aneurin Bevan, faced considerable opposition to his proposals, especially from the British Medical Association (BMA) and from many Conservative MPs.

- The BMA opposed the changes – a survey of its members in January 1948 showed that 90 per cent of its members would refuse to cooperate with the NHS.
- Many local authorities and voluntary bodies opposed the nationalisation of all hospitals, fearing they would lose control over them.
- Arguments raged over the enormous costs involved.

However, Bevan was able to win the arguments by agreeing to a compromise which allowed doctors to take on fee-paying patients as long as they treated NHS patients as well. By the spring of 1948 opposition had crumbled and by the time the NHS was officially launched on 5 July 1948 over 90 per cent of doctors had enrolled on the new scheme.

> **Source O:** An extract from a speech made by Aneurin Bevan, Minister for Health, in 1946
>
> *Medical treatment should be made available to rich and poor alike in accordance with medical need and no other criteria. Worry about money in a time of sickness is a serious hindrance to recovery apart from its unnecessary cruelty. The records show that it is the mother in the average family who suffers most from the absence of a full health service. In trying to balance her budget she puts her own needs last. No society can call itself civilised if a sick person is denied medical aid because of lack of [money]. The essence of a satisfactory health service is that the rich and the poor are treated alike, that poverty is not a disability, and wealth is not advantaged.*

> **Source P:** An extract from the *British Medical Journal*, 18 January 1946
>
> *If the Bill is passed no patient or doctor will feel safe from interference by some ministerial edict or regulation. The Minister's spies will be everywhere, and intrigue will rule.*

> **THINK**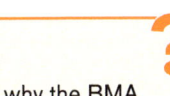
>
> 1. Explain why the BMA was initially opposed to the setting up of an NHS.
> 2. Study Source O. What arguments does Aneurin Bevan put forward to support his idea of creating a national health service?

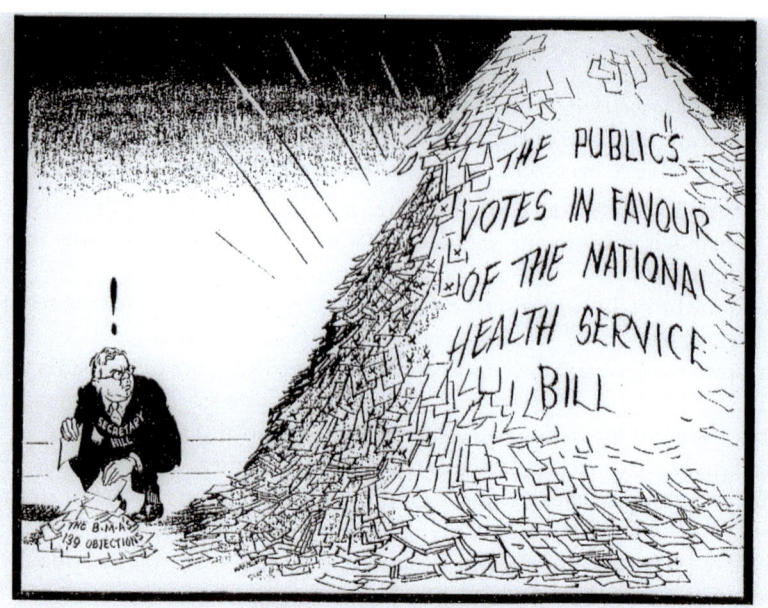

Hill meets mountain!

Source Q: A cartoon published in the *Daily Mirror* in 1946, suggesting that Bevan's proposals to create a NHS were popular

> **Source R:** An account which appeared in the *Daily Mail* on 5 July 1948, the day the NHS officially came into being
>
> *On Monday morning you will wake in a New Britain, a state which takes over its citizens six months before they are born, providing care and free services from their birth, their schooling, sickness, workless days, widowhood and retirement. Finally, it helps [pay] the costs of their departure. All this, with free doctoring, dentistry and medicine – free bath chairs, too, if needed – for 4s. 11d [25p] of your weekly pay packet.*

In October 1949 Bevan quoted figures to show what use had been made of the NHS since its launch the previous July:

- 187 million prescriptions had been written out
- 5.2 million pairs of glasses had been issued
- 8.5 million people had received free dental treatment

By 1951 only 1.5 per cent of the population remained outside the NHS and when the Conservative government took office that year it agreed to keep the NHS.

Development of the NHS since 1948

The NHS is a very costly service to run and during its 68-year history there have been attempts to introduce changes. Demand for healthcare was huge, much greater than expected. In 1950 the NHS budget was under pressure and in 1952 charges for spectacles were introduced, prescriptions cost 1 shilling (5p) and dental treatment £1. It was the end of a completely free NHS.

Other changes occurred over the following decades:
- In the early 1960s a new building programme was begun to replace out-of-date hospitals.
- The Thatcher governments (1979–90) tried to cut the cost of the NHS and encouraged people to pay for private medical care.
- During the 1990s hospitals were allowed to become trusts and GPs were allowed to become fund holders, buying services from hospitals and other providers.
- In 1998 NHS Direct was launched, providing 24-hour health advice over the phone.
- In 2002 primary care trusts were launched to allow for the administration and delivery of healthcare at the local level.
- In 2004 foundation trusts were launched, run by local managers, staff and members of the public.

> **THINK**
>
> 1. Use Source R and your own knowledge to describe the key features of the NHS when it was launched in 1948.
> 2. How has the NHS changed since 1948 to reflect the demands made upon a modern health service?

5 Developments in patient care

FOCUS TASK REVISITED

As you have worked through this chapter you have completed a time chart which has outlined the key developments in hospital, nursing and patient care. This will have provided you with an overview of the key changes, when they occurred, why they occurred and the impact they had. It is important that you use this fact file to build up a picture of the developments in patient care across time.

Use your time chart to identify:

1 which periods witnessed the most dramatic change in the functions and layout of hospitals
2 which periods witnessed the most dramatic change in the standards of nursing and patient care
3 the reasons why these changes occurred when they did.

ACTIVITY

What evidence can you find to support the view that since the beginning of the twentieth century the government has increasingly replaced voluntary organisations as the most important body responsible for providing care for patients?

TOPIC SUMMARY

- In medieval times the church played the principal role in providing hospital facilities and administering patient care.
- Patients entered medieval hospitals not to be cured of their illness but to receive God's protection and to pray and attend religious services.
- The dissolution of the monasteries in the mid-sixteenth century had a major impact upon the care of patients as the church no longer played such an active role.
- During the sixteenth and seventeenth centuries voluntary organisations began to take on the role of setting up and funding hospitals and patient care.
- These tended to be established in large towns and cities, and some came to specialise in the care of particular types of patients.
- During the eighteenth century there was a big expansion in the number of hospitals being built, financed through endowments by wealthy individuals.
- While new hospitals were built, the quality of nursing remained poor, as did the conditions for patients.
- The Crimean War helped change nursing care and this was largely the result of the actions of one woman, Florence Nightingale.
- Nightingale established new standards in nursing and patient care; she turned nursing into a respected profession.
- During the early twentieth century the government began to take on responsibility for the welfare of its people, setting up a National Insurance scheme to provide free medical treatment to those who paid into the scheme.
- The key turning point for national state care was the Beveridge Report of 1942 which recommended the government take action to establish a national system of free medical care.
- The result was the creation of the National Health Service in 1948 which offered free medical care to all from 'the cradle to the grave'.

Practice questions

1 Explain why the church played an important part in caring for sick people during the medieval period. *(For guidance, see page 126.)*
2 Explain why 'royal endowments' were so important in the provision of care for sick and poor people in London after the mid-sixteenth century. *(For guidance, see page 126.)*
3 Describe the growth of endowed voluntary hospitals during the eighteenth century. *(For guidance, see page 125.)*
4 Study Source C (page 69), Source D (page 69) and Source E (page 70). Use these three sources to identify one similarity and one difference in the care of patients in hospital over time. *(For guidance, see page 121.)*
5 Explain why the Crimean War played an important part in the development of professional nursing care. *(For guidance, see page 126.)*
6 Study Sources Q and R. Which of the two sources is the more reliable to a historian studying the establishment of the National Health Service? *(For guidance, see page 123.)*
7 Outline how standards of patient care have improved from c.500 to the present day. *(For guidance, see page 127.)*

6 Developments in public health and welfare

This chapter focuses on the key question: How effective were attempts to improve public health and welfare over time?

Throughout history people have tried to keep themselves clean and healthy, not always successfully. There have also always been attempts by town councils and governments to pass laws to clean up nuisances, keep drinking water clean, and so on. But how successful have they been? Were medieval people, for example, dirtier than Victorian people? And if the measures used to improve public health *have* been successful, why do so many people still live in unhealthy conditions? This chapter explores the developments in public health and welfare over the last 1000 years or so.

FOCUS TASK

1. In the nineteenth century people wanting to reform public health became known as the 'Clean Party', whereas those opposed to it were called the 'Dirty Party'. As you work through *each* section of this chapter make a list, like the one below, of actions that might have been, or were, proposed by the Clean Party, that is, those wanting change; and why they were proposed. The first one has been done for you as an example.

The Clean Party	
Action	Reason
1388 Act of Parliament	To clear away nuisances in the streets

2. Similarly, compile a list of actions that were, or might have been, proposed by the Dirty Party.

The Dirty Party	
Action	Reason

You will need these lists when you have finished studying the chapter.

Public health and hygiene in medieval society

In the medieval period it was said you could smell a town long before you could see it. In Exeter, for example, you entered the town by a bridge crossing a river known locally as 'Shitebrook', where the night-soil men dumped their waste into the river. Mortality was higher in the towns and cities than in the countryside. People lived closer together, alongside their animals and their filth. We have already seen in Chapter 1 how unhealthy towns and cities were to live in. But were all towns and cities the same?

THINK

Look at Source A. Identify all the health hazards you can find in this picture of a medieval town.

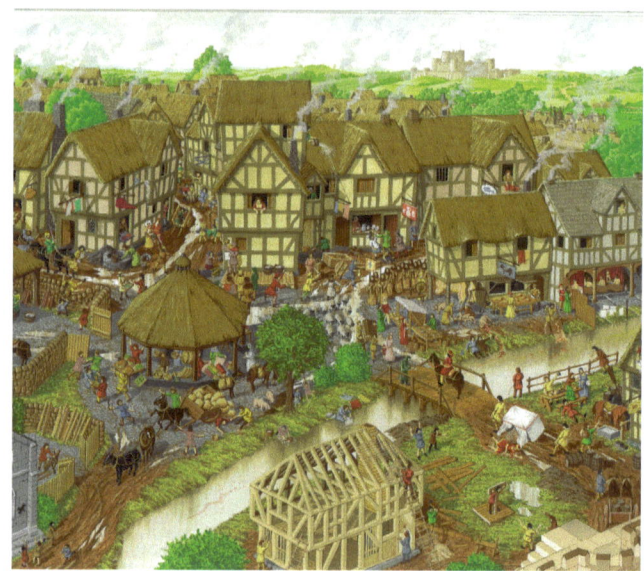

▲ **Source A:** A modern interpetation of a medieval town

A case study of Coventry: were all medieval towns dirty and unhealthy places to live?

Surprisingly, the answer to this question is 'no'. Historian Dolly Jorgensen, in a recent academic paper 'What to do with waste', argues convincingly that Coventry council made a concerted and consistent effort to clean up the city.

In 1421 the mayor's proclamation required that every man clean the street in front of his house every Saturday or pay a 12 penny fine, with no exceptions being made. Waste collection services are recorded in 1420, when the council gave William Oteley the right to collect 1 penny from every resident and shop, on a quarterly basis, for his weekly street cleansing and waste removal services. The waste was to be sold to nearby farmers.

The council also specified designated waste disposal locations. Dunghills and waste pits naturally sprang up around the perimeter of the town. The council authorised the use of specific sites for particular types of waste. By 1427, five designated waste-disposal locations are mentioned for Coventry (Dolly Jorgenson only specifically lists four):

- a dunghill outside of the city limit beyond Greyfriar Gate
- a pit in the Little Park Street Gate
- a muckhill near the cross situated beyond New Gate, at Derne Gate
- a pit at Poodycroft.

In total, Coventry's council banned waste disposal in the River Sherbourne nine times between 1421 and 1475. There are, of course, two ways of looking at this. That the council took action, and it was widely ignored. Or, perhaps, the actions worked and when one or two individuals went back to the old ways then residents complained to the council who then took action.

In 1421 all latrines over the Red Ditch, a local stream, were ordered to be removed, to allow free flowing of the water, and to prevent flooding. Attempts were made to stop local stables and butchers throwing waste into the River Sherbourne, again to prevent flooding. All this evidence shows active intervention by the mayor and corporation of Coventry when faced with complaints by residents about the state of the town.

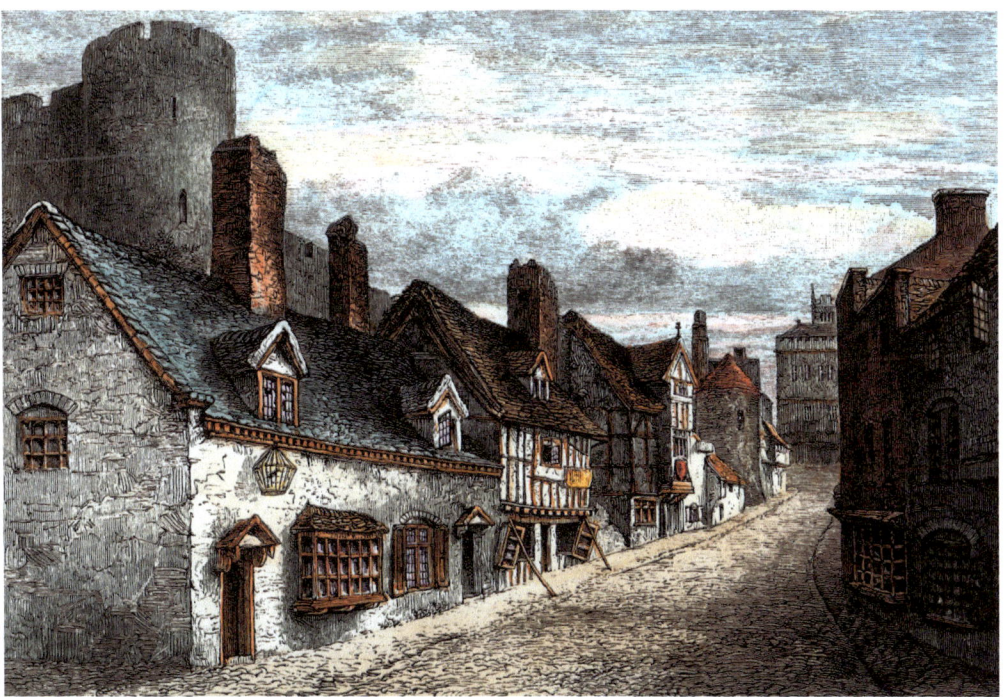

▲ **Source B:** Some towns, such as Shrewsbury shown here, made efforts to become clean and orderly

THINK

1. Does Dolly Jorgenson's paper on Coventry (she uses York as an example too) prove that towns were cleaner than we think?
2. What other actions could Coventry have taken to clean itself up?
3. How significant is the case of Coventry in understanding how clean British towns were at this time?
4. Which source best reflects Coventry as described by Dolly Jorgenson, Source A or Source B? Which source do you think is more realistic? Why?

Public health and hygiene in the sixteenth and seventeenth centuries

Look back at the weekly 'bill of mortality' for London for the week 21–28 February 1664 (Source E, page 22). How healthy was London as a place to live in 1664? There were outbreaks of the plague in 1563 (when 17,000 people were said to have died in London), 1575, 1584, 1589, 1603, 1636, 1647 and of course the biggest outbreak of all in 1665. In Aberdeen in 1647 the corporation passed regulations to control the plague including 'poysonne laid for destroying mice and rattons'. Towns and cities were still incredibly dirty and unhealthy places to live.

Yet there had been some attempts to improve public health. Henry VII recognised the menace to health from slaughterhouses and passed a law forbidding them within cities or towns, 'leste it might engendre sicknes, unto the destruction of the people'. In 1532 Henry VIII passed an act of parliament giving towns and cities the power to impose a tax in order to build sewers. Few places did. In 1547 people were forbidden to go to the toilet in the courtyards of the Royal Palaces – they had to find somewhere else to relieve themselves. Elizabeth I is said to have had a bath once every month of her life. Samuel Pepys states in his diary, in 1666, that his wife Elizabeth refused to allow him into the marriage bed until he had washed and had a bath. People were clearly making the link between dirt and disease. Yet towns and cities, and especially London, were growing so fast it was impossible to keep them clean.

After the Great Fire of London in 1666 an act of parliament was passed. 'An Act for the rebuilding of London ... and for the better regulation, uniformity and gracefulness of such new buildings as shall be erected for habitations', was designed to limit fire destruction by making streets wider, by insisting houses were built of stone with tile or slate roofs. Some historians argue that the rebuilding of London after the fire made it a healthier place, yet in 1690 we get yet another act of parliament requiring the paving and cleaning of the streets in London and surrounding areas, followed by further acts over the next few years requiring the removal of dung and the cleansing of common stairways, and prohibiting the keeping of pigs in dwelling houses.

> ### THINK
> 1. 'Medieval towns were relatively clean compared to the sixteenth and seventeenth centuries'. How far do you agree with this statement?
> 2. How similar were attempts to clean up medieval Coventry and those of the sixteenth and seventeenth century?
> 3. In what way does Source C reinforce the view that London was an unhealthy place in which to live?

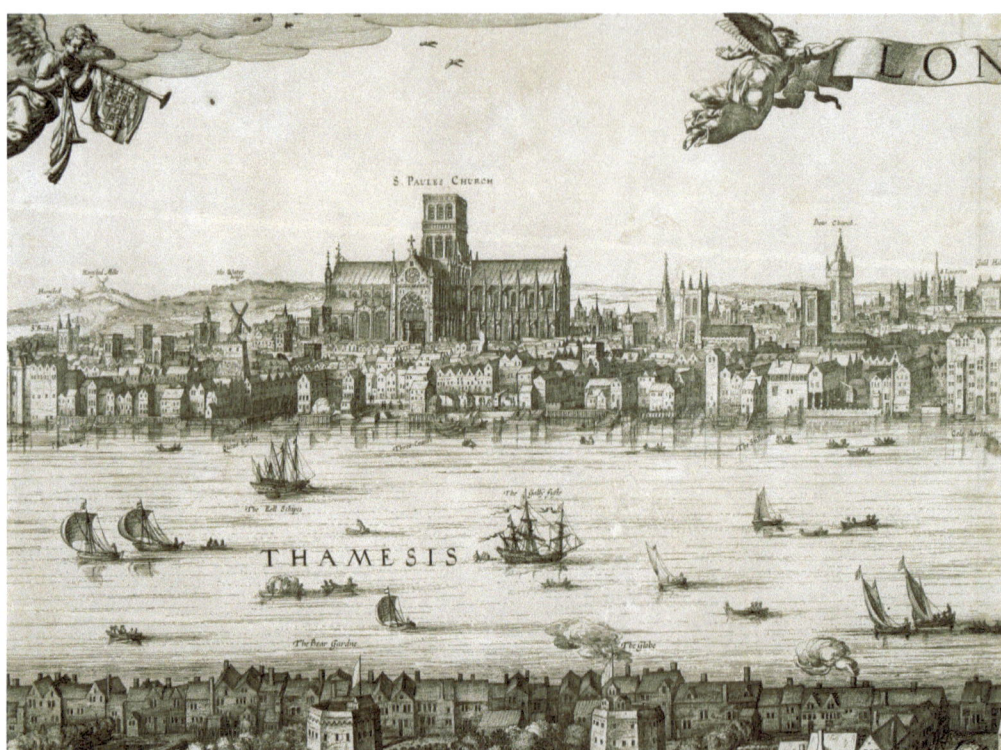

Source C: Etching by Wenceslaus Hollar, a Czech artist living and working in London, c.1653. It shows part of London before the Great Fire of London

6 Developments in public health and welfare

The impact of industrialisation on public health in the nineteenth century

In the nineteenth century many people moved to the cities to live (see Table 6.1). This is where the jobs were. Manchester made cotton, Birmingham made metal goods, Bradford spun and wove woollen cloth, Stoke on Trent made pottery, all in the new workshops and factories. By 1851 more people lived in towns than in the country, and Britain was known as the 'Workshop of the World'. Britain became rich making things and exporting them to the rest of the world.

People had to live close to where they worked, and there were very few building regulations. The supply of water, gas, and later electricity was all left to private companies who needed to make a profit, so areas where there were better-off people might have good supplies, whereas areas of poor people were not well served. As we have already seen in Chapter 5, the government believed in the philosophy of laissez-faire or 'leave it alone' meaning it was not the government's job to regulate things like working conditions, houses, transport and the like – it was up to individuals to do that for themselves. As a result working-class housing in the industrial cities could be very poor (see Sources D and E). In 1842 the average age of death for a member of a labourer's family in rural Rutland was 38; in Manchester, it was 17. And we have already seen in Chapter 1 that in Bethnal Green, in London, it was 16.

Town	1801	1851	1901
London	957,000	2,362,000	4,536,000
Birmingham	71,000	233,000	523,000
Manchester	70,409	303,000	645,000
Liverpool	82,000	376,000	704,000
Bradford	13,000	104,000	280,000
Cardiff	2,000	18,000	164,000

▲ Table 6.1: Town growth, 1801–1901

Source E: From *'The Victorian Underworld'*, Kellow Chesney

Hideous slums, some of them acres wide, some no more than crannies of obscure misery, make up a substantial part of the metropolis [London] ... In big, once handsome houses, thirty or more people of all ages may inhabit a single room.

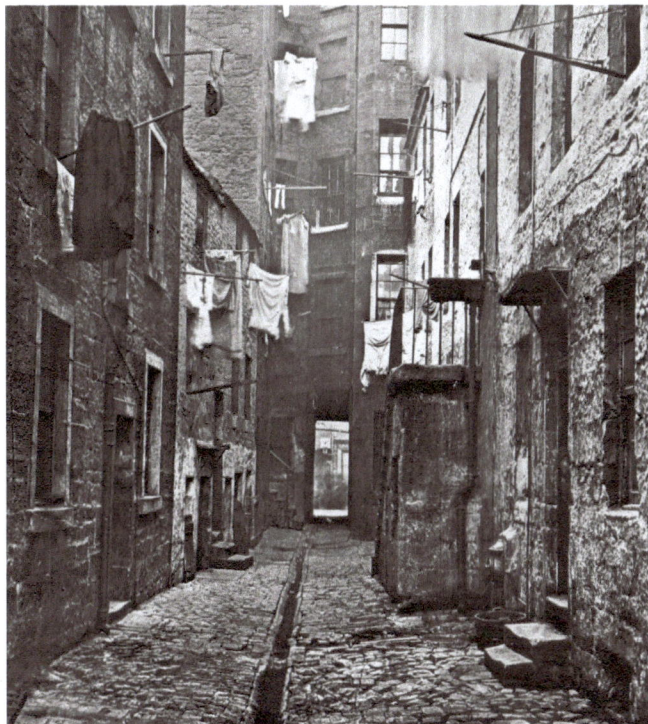

◀ **Source D:** A Glasgow slum, 1868

THINK

1. Look at Table 6.1 What problems might such rapid growth of towns and cities cause for public health and welfare?
2. Look at Source D. What might it have been like to live in one of these houses? How might you keep yourself and your family clean, warm and dry?
3. To what extent does the interpretation of towns in Source E reflect both Table 6.1 and Source E in its portrayal of Victorian cities?
4. What evidence do you think Chesney has used to make his interpretation? Do you know any evidence he might have used that might have changed his interpretation to give a better view of Victorian cities?

The work of Edwin Chadwick leading to Victorian improvements in public health

In 1854 a letter to *The Times* newspaper stated, 'We prefer to take our chance with cholera rather than be bullied into health.' This epitomises the great struggle that took place in the nineteenth century to persuade the government to act over living and working conditions. Edwin Chadwick was a member of the Poor Law Commission, set up as a consequence of the Poor Law Reform Act 1834. He became convinced that most people were poor because of ill-health rather than idleness, and spent the rest of his life advocating improvements in public health. He published his influential 'Report on the Sanitary Conditions of the Labouring Population' in 1842. Chadwick was instrumental in setting up the Health of Towns Association in 1844, which led to the first Public Health Act in 1848. This was the first time that the government had legislated on health issues.

Chadwick was an influential member of what became known as the 'Clean Party'. The Clean Party were those pushing for government action to improve conditions in towns. The 'Dirty Party', as they became known, were those MPs and others opposed to any such action. Their opposition was largely based on the monumental costs involved. Ratepayers, the wealthier people in a town, were keen to keep their rates (local taxes used to pay for local government) as low as possible so they favoured inaction. It was a member of the Dirty Party that wrote the 1854 letter to *The Times*.

> **THINK**
> 1. What part did Chadwick play in improving public health in the nineteenth century?
> 2. Why was the debate over reform referred to as the 'Clean Party versus the Dirty Party'?

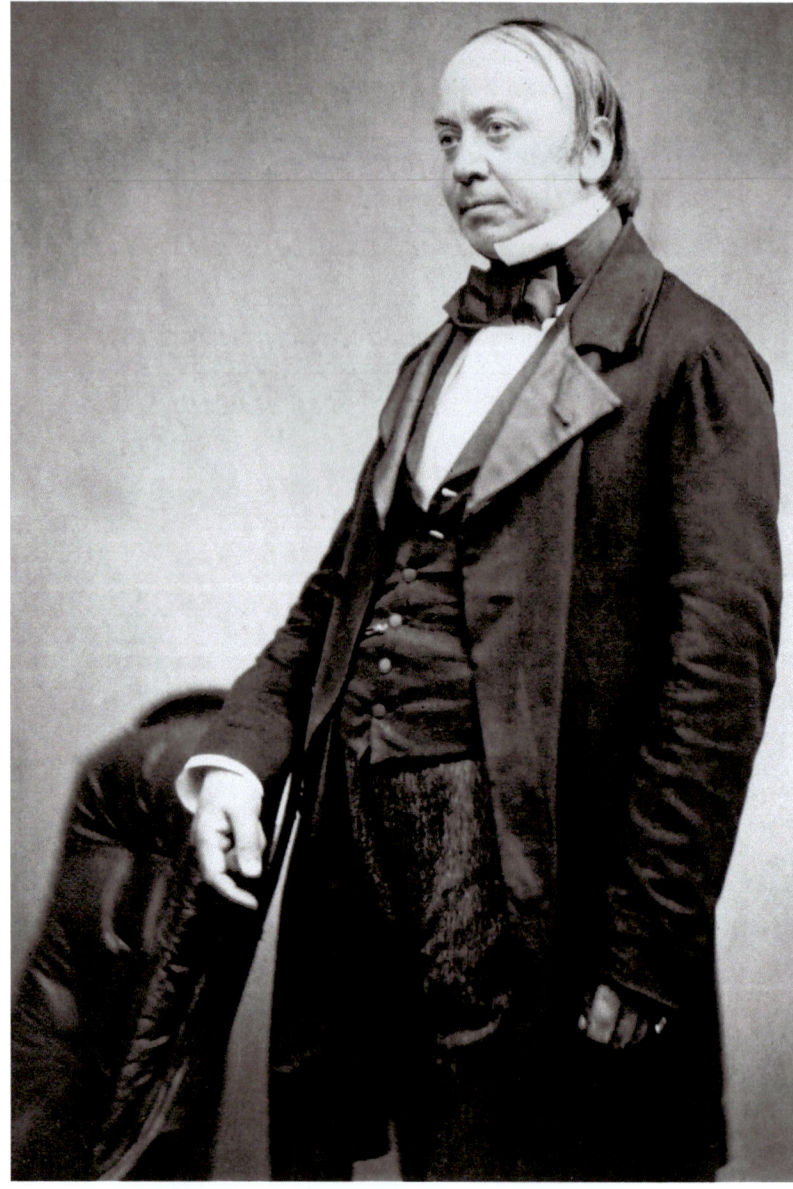

▲ Edwin Chadwick, *c.*1854, physician and social reformer

6 Developments in public health and welfare

The government acts at last: the great clean-up

It was the cholera epidemic of 1848, which killed over 52,000 people in England, rather than the Health of Towns Association that finally forced the government to act. They passed the Public Health Act 1848. This allowed local councils to improve conditions in their own town *if* they wished, and if they were prepared to pay for it. They could force towns with a particularly high death rate to take action over water supply and sewage, and to appoint a medical officer of health. The Central Board of Health was created and although it was abolished ten years later, the Act also encouraged local boards of health to be set up to appoint a medical officer, provide sewers, inspect lodging houses and check food which was offered for sale.

It was a start, but by 1872 only 50 councils had a medical officer of health. Some towns, like Leeds, took steps to improve their facilities, but many did not. Other acts followed, such as the Sanitary Act 1866, the Artisans Dwellings Act 1875 and finally the Public Health Act 1875, which was the real breakthrough. This Act had more power. It brought together a range of acts covering sewerage and drains, water supply, housing and disease. Local councils were *forced* to provide clean water, and appoint medical officers of health and sanitary inspectors who were to look after slaughterhouses and prevent contaminated food being sold. Local authorities were ordered to cover sewers, keep them in good condition, supply fresh water to their citizens, collect rubbish and provide street lighting. The Food and Drugs Act 1875 even regulated food and medicines. *Laissez-faire* seemed banished, as government began to take responsibility for public health.

London started building new sewers in 1858, and without doubt new sewers improved living conditions and public health. But there were other contributing factors. The Housing Act 1875 allowed councils to knock down poor housing and replace it. Flush toilets became more widely used in better-off homes and new products, like Pear's soap, became available and were cheap, making it easier for people and clothes to stay clean.

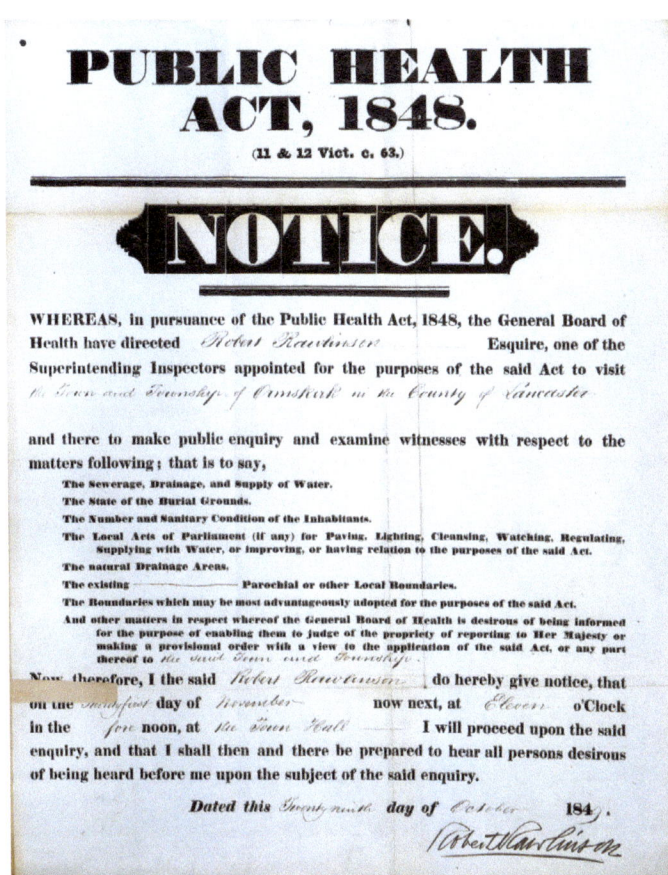

Source F: A poster that appeared in the town of Ormskirk in Lancashire in October 1848. It was signed by the inspector appointed for Ormskirk

THINK

1. What does Source F announce? What is going to happen in November 1848? On whose authority?
2. What does the poster tell us about the Public Health Act 1848?
3. Does this poster prove that the Public Health Act 1848 was effective at improving public health in Ormskirk? In Lancashire? In Britain? Explain your answer.

Case study: Sir Titus Salt – an individual acts to improve public health

Titus Salt was born near Leeds and moved to Bradford to work with his father as a woolstapler (wool dealer). He used Donskoi wool from Russia, alpaca fleece from South America and Mohair from angora goats in Turkey to make fine quality worsted cloths. By 1850 he owned and ran five separate spinning and weaving mills in Bradford and was the biggest employer in the area. His firm exhibited at the Great Exhibition in 1851, and sent cloth throughout the world. Queen Victoria was a customer for his alpaca cloth. Bradford had grown very rapidly, from 13,000 in 1803 to 43,000 in 1833 and over 100,000 in 1851. Conditions were very poor. One visitor in 1846, a German named George Weerth, wrote home, 'every other town in England is a paradise compared to this hole'. There were over 200 factory chimneys belching out smoke every day. Life expectancy for the poor at this time in Bradford was 20 years. Cholera and other diseases frequently broke out in the cramped conditions.

In 1843 a local man, Lister, invented a wool-combing machine and thousands of wool combers soon found themselves unemployed. Titus Salt set up and paid for soup kitchens to help. He was chosen as the second mayor of Bradford in 1848 and tried to persuade the council and local factory owners to do something to improve living and working conditions in Bradford. He failed. He even paid for his 2000 workers to have a day out in the country using the newly opened railway. In 1850 Salt took the decision to move his factories out of Bradford and bought a site at Shipley, out in the country but adjacent to the railway, the Leeds and Liverpool Canal, and the River Aire. Here, he built the largest and most up-to-date mill in Europe. The mill opened in 1853 employing 3500 workers.

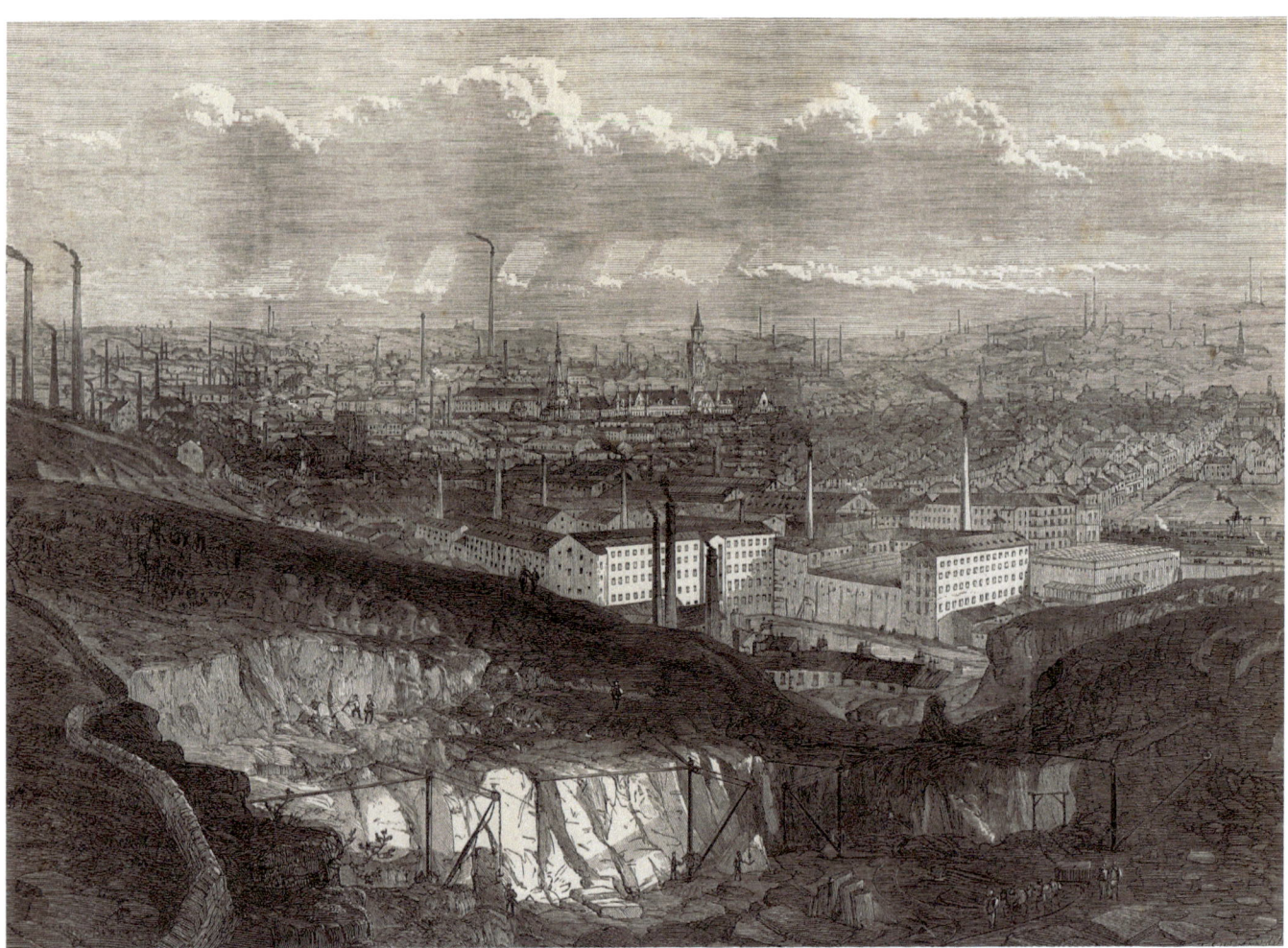

▲ **Source G:** Bradford 1873 engraving, view from Cliff Quarry

Saltaire

Not only did Salt build a mill, he also built a model village for his workers and called it Saltaire. His 11 children all had streets in the village named after them. There were over 800 houses (but no pubs) as well as wash houses with running water; bath houses; a hospital; an institute containing reading rooms, a library, a billiard room, a science lab and a concert hall; a school; a church; almshouses; allotments; a park; and a boathouse. He also donated land for a Methodist chapel to be built. He said he built the village 'to do good, and give his sons employment'. Saltaire is regarded as one of the best examples of nineteenth-century urban planning and is now a World Heritage Site.

Salt's motives

Historians argue about Salt's motives for building Saltaire. He claimed it was to help his workers lead 'healthy, virtuous lives'. Some say it was a matter of simple economics. Here he could control his workers better, and run his factories longer. It was also built beside the Leeds–Liverpool canal (visible in Source H) making it easy to move materials in and out. Others argued that it allowed Salt to show off his power and wealth. Another possible motive was tied up with his religious beliefs; that it was his Christian duty to try to make things better for those less fortunate than himself. When he died in 1876 an estimated 100,000 people lined the streets of Bradford to watch his funeral procession. The editor of the *Bradford Observer* wrote: 'Sir Titus Salt was perhaps the greatest captain of industry in England, not only because he gathered thousands under him, but also because, according to the light that was in him, he tried to care for all those thousands … he was upright in business, admirable in his private relations, he came without seeking the honour to be admittedly the best representative of the Employer Class in this part of the Country if not the whole Kingdom.'

> **THINK**
> 1. Look carefully at Sources G and H. Would you prefer to live in Bradford, or in Saltaire? Why?
> 2. Were the workers in Saltaire better off or worse off than they had been in Bradford?
> 3. Why do you think Titus Salt built a model village for his workers?
> 4. What does the life of Titus Salt tell us about public health in nineteenth-century Britain?

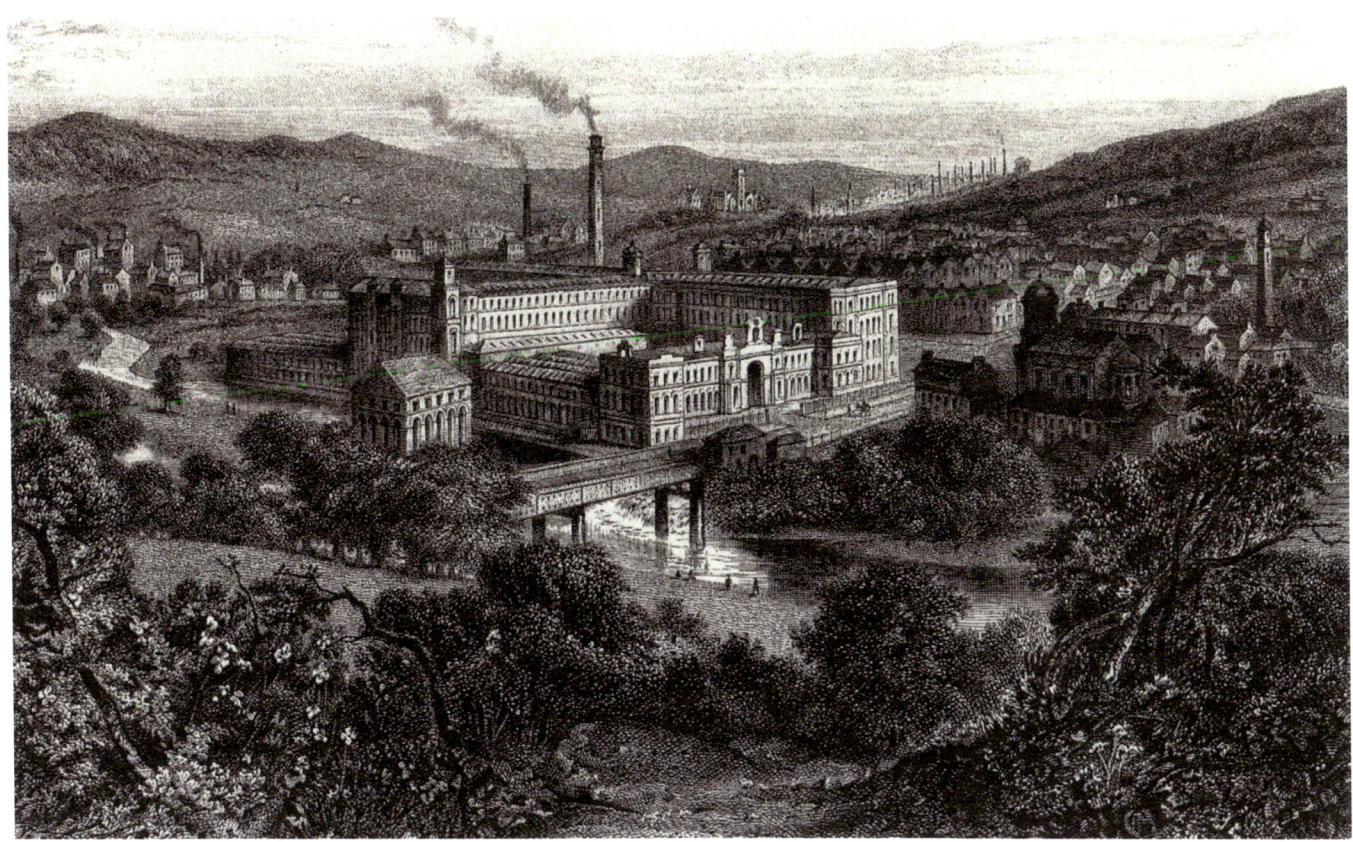

▲ Source H: Saltaire – engraving from *c.*1860

Birmingham and 'municipal socialism': a town acts to improve public health

As we have seen, throughout the 1840s and 1850s there was a gradual increase in local and central government intervention in public health, albeit reluctantly and always within the philosophy of voluntarism – even the 1848 Public Health Act allowed councils to improve conditions *if they wished*.

Birmingham provides an interesting case study of a local council that finally grasped the nettle of public health improvement. In the 1840s and 1850s the council was controlled by ratepayers who resisted demands to spend money. They blocked a move to purchase the Birmingham Waterworks Company (it was too expensive) and dismissed the borough engineer, replacing him immediately with his deputy at half the salary. They cut spending on roads by 50 per cent. In consequence, according to Thomas Carlyle, 'the streets are ill-built, ill-paved, always flimsy in their aspect – often poor, sometimes miserable. Not above one or two of them are paved with flagstones at the side.' The editor of the *Birmingham Daily Post* declared that citizens were so ashamed of their city that they refused to show the town centre to their visitors.

All that changed when Joseph Chamberlain became mayor in 1873. He devised what he called 'gas and water socialism', whereby the council would take over the gas and water companies, improve supplies, and use the profits to make the city a better place to live. He persuaded the council to borrow £2 million to buy the gas companies in 1875. By 1879 the council had made £165,000 profit to spend on other projects, and built a public park on ten acres of derelict gas company land. By 1884 they had also reduced gas prices by 30 per cent. Water followed in 1876, and by 1880 the death rate in central Birmingham had dropped from 25.2 per thousand to 20.7 per thousand. The council also obtained a Birmingham Improvement Act in 1876 allowing it to clear 40 acres of slums in the centre of the city, removing 9000 people in the process, and replace these slums with a shopping centre (another source of income for the council), a council house, an art gallery, public library and new, broad, well-paved streets. Chamberlain wrote, in a letter to a friend in June 1876, that 'I think I have now almost completed my municipal programme. The town will be parked, paved, assised [magistrates courts], marketed, Gas-and-Watered and improved – all as the result of three years' active work.'

THINK

1. How had attitudes to public health in Birmingham changed between the 1840s and the 1880s?
2. What was 'municipal socialism?' How did it work in Birmingham?
3. Do you think public health in Birmingham had improved by 1886?
4. Source I was published in 1886, at the time of the improvements in Birmingham. Does that make it reliable?
5. Which do you think had the most impact in Birmingham – the Public Health Act 1875 or Joseph Chamberlain? Why?

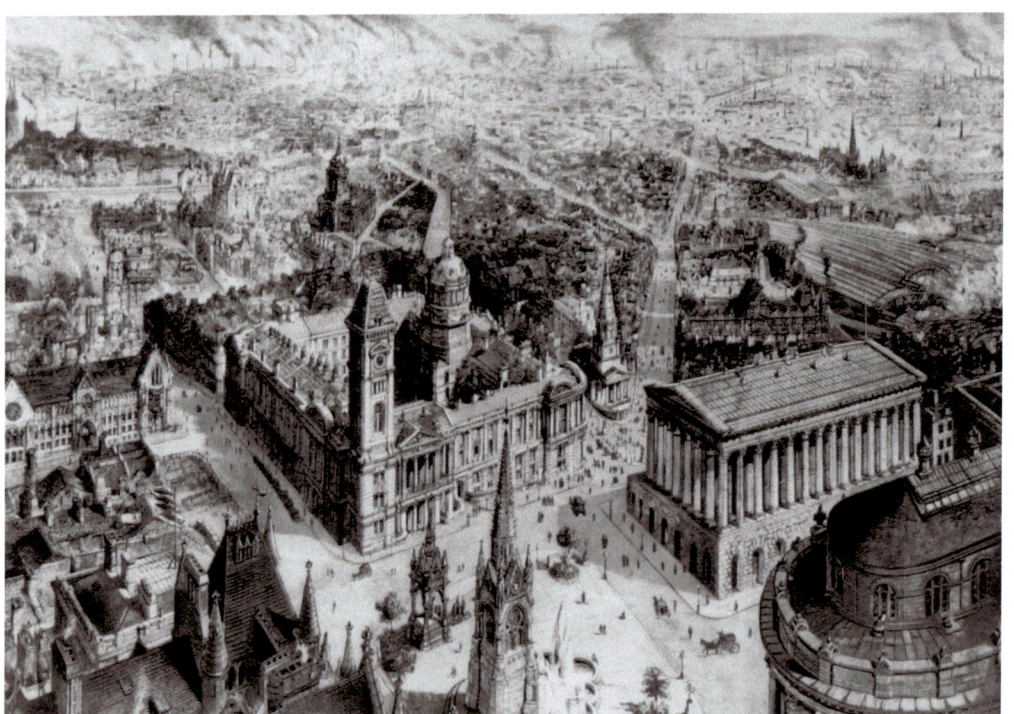

Source I: A drawing by H.W. Brewer, taken from *The Graphic*, 1886. It shows Birmingham city centre in 1886 looking over Chamberlain Square with the newly extended council house and art gallery (in the centre), the town hall (the building with pillars on the right) and Christ Church between them

Efforts to improve housing and pollution in the twentieth century

The twentieth century has seen a major shift in the role of government with regards to public health. The Victorian *laissez-faire* attitude has been replaced by an acceptance that it is the role of government to ensure people live healthy lives, but the extent of that role is still open to debate even today.

Identifying the problem

When the Boer War broke out in 1899, many volunteers for the army were unfit to serve. This was a shock to people at the time, and led to worries about the continued growth of the economy and strength of the British Empire. The state of these volunteers for the army provided the inspiration to investigate living conditions and the health of ordinary people in the new industrial cities, which eventually led to the changes introduced by the Liberal government from 1906. As a result, some social surveys were carried out in order to understand the extent of the problem. Charles Booth, in his *Life and Labour of the People* published in 1889 found that 35 per cent of London's population were living in abject poverty. His detailed survey had originally been designed to prove that the belief that 25 per cent of the population lived in poverty was far too high.

Seebohm Rowntree was inspired by Booth's work to do the same in York, where he lived. In 1897 and 1898 his researchers interviewed over 46,000 citizens of York, and his results were published in *Poverty, A Study in Town Life*, in 1901. He found that very nearly one-half of the working-class people in York lived in poverty. He is acknowledged as the inventor of the term 'poverty line', and became an adviser to the British Liberal politician Lloyd George after 1906.

A third book played an influential part in shifting opinion. In 1913 Maud Pember Reeves published *Round About a Pound A Week*, a detailed study of the way workers, many of them in regular employment like policemen, struggled to exist on an average wage of £1 a week. She had set out to prove that these families wasted money on drink but found that often women were going without food so the man (the wage earner) and the children could eat.

Progress after the First World War

The Housing Act 1919 proposed to build 500,000 homes 'Fit for Heroes', as the slogan at the time stated, but only half were built. Throughout the 1920s and 1930s there were subsidies for building council houses to rent to workers, and acts of parliament encouraging the demolition of slum properties, but economic difficulties between the wars limited progress. These were the first generation of houses to feature electricity, running water, bathrooms, indoor toilets and front and rear gardens. However, until well into the 1930s, some were being built with outdoor toilets. By 1939 over 1 million houses had been built by councils for workers to live in, but nearly 3 million had been built for better-off families. The damage and destruction during the Second World War made the demand for 'affordable' housing even greater. Clement Attlee's Labour government of 1945–51 built another 1 million homes. In the 1950s and 1960s emphasis changed to slum clearance from city centres.

> **THINK**
> 1 Why were *Life and Labour of the People*, *Poverty, A Study in Town Life* and *Round About a Pound A Week* so influential at the time?
> 2 How similar, and how different, are the problems identified by the authors of these three books to those identified by Edwin Chadwick and Thomas Southwood Smith (page 84)?

Clean air, new towns and tower blocks: the definitive answer to public health?

In December 1952, London was engulfed in what became known as the 'Killer Smog'. Air pollution and fumes from coal fires were trapped by an anticyclone over the city from 5–9 December. Recent estimates suggest over 12,000 people died and as many as 100,000 were taken ill as a result. It was the worst example of air pollution in Britain and led to the government passing Clean Air Acts in 1956 and 1968. This encouraged householders throughout the country to change from coal fires to the cleaner gas and electricity, or even burn coke and other smokeless fuels. There were further attempts to improve air quality in the Environment Protection Act 1990 and the Clean Air Act 1993. Both of these were focused on 'greenhouse gas' issues and aimed to limit both factory and motor car emissions. Latest research still shows that up to 27,000 people each year die prematurely from the impact of air pollution. Air pollution is an on going issue in many cities.

New towns and cities were also developed, such as Milton Keynes and Telford, in an attempt to move people out of dirty, overcrowded neighbourhoods into 'greener' settings, with industry and housing carefully segregated from one other. The first new town, at Letchworth, was the work of Ebenezer Howard, in 1903. Housing was meant to be attractive and spacious, gardens were an integral part of the plan, as were public parks and amenities. Cycle routes and pedestrian walkways were separated from traffic, to make it safer for all. By 2014 over 2.7 million people lived in new towns or cities in the UK.

In the 1960s, slum clearance took place in old towns and cities too, with a massive expansion of council-built housing in an attempt to provide everyone with a decent home to live in. Unfit housing was demolished and often replaced with 'modern' tower blocks; high-rise blocks of flats with all modern conveniences like central heating, bathrooms and fitted kitchens.

Towns like Chelmsley Wood, just outside Birmingham, sprung up overnight. From 1965 it was created on a greenfield site, with over 16,000 houses designed to house 50,000 people who were unable to find a home in the city. At the time it was the largest single residential development in Europe. Cumbernauld, just outside Glasgow, is another new town, started in 1956, and it is now the eighth largest town in Scotland.

Public reaction to the new towns is often mixed. Cumbernauld town centre, for example, was voted 'the worst building in Britain' in 2005, yet it was voted the 'Best Town' in Scotland in 2012. The new tower blocks were often built cheaply, from concrete and on out-of-town 'greenfield' sites. People usually liked the interiors, but often found themselves isolated from their community, missing their neighbours, the local shops and the pub on the street corner. Poor maintenance and cheap construction have led to many of these 'ideal' homes in the sky being demolished as people simply did not want to live in them.

ACTIVITIES

1. Carry out your own research on a new town that has been proposed or is being built near where you live.
2. How is it similar, and how is it different, to the new towns of the 1960s?

THINK

Why do you think so much emphasis was placed on building better housing for people?

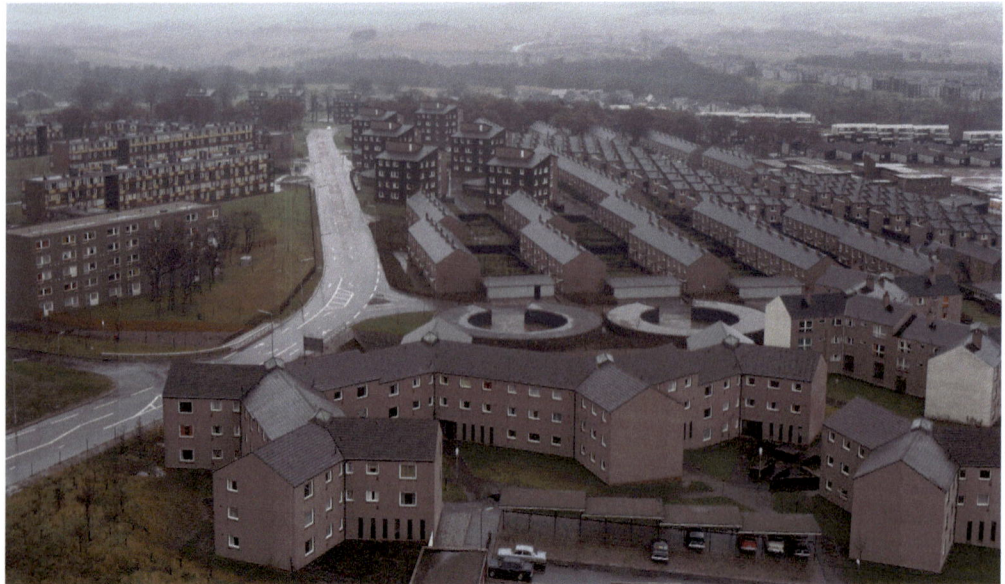

◀ Source J: View of new town housing in Cumbernauld, 1970, built to solve the severe shortage of housing in post-war Glasgow

6 Developments in public health and welfare

Local and national government attempts to improve public health and welfare in the twenty-first century: campaigns, fitness drives, healthy eating

Unhealthy lifestyles?

It seems stories such as the one in Source K appear in the news nearly every day. Scientists estimate that many of us are reducing our life expectancy by our lifestyle. We eat too much, often of the wrong foods, drink too much alcohol, do not take enough exercise and smoke too much. We also spend too much time sitting at a desk or playing computer games rather than exercising. All this adds up to a recipe for obesity and ill health. Obesity is one of the greatest causes of heart disease. So despite better diagnoses of illness, the availability of more effective medicines and skilled surgeons, it is all to no avail if we refuse to follow a healthy lifestyle.

> **Source K:** *Daily Telegraph*, 28 September 2015
>
> *Just one can of fizzy drink a day can increase the risk of heart attack by a third and dramatically raise the chance of diabetes and stroke, the largest ever study has found. The study ... follows new official UK advice which says adults should restrict their sugar intake to just 30 grams – seven teaspoons – a day.*

Prevention or cure?

Throughout the twentieth century and today in the twenty-first century, governments have put more and more effort into health education, trying to persuade people to live healthier lifestyles and look after themselves better. Some people argue it is not the job of the government to do this; remember the letter to *The Times* newspaper at the time of the cholera outbreak in 1854 (see page 84)? Some people still think like that, arguing it is up to each individual to make their own choices. Others argue that there is a cost associated with poor lifestyle choices. For example, if people stopped smoking this would save the NHS millions of pounds each year. As fewer people would get sick, they would miss less time off work, and so it would also help the country get richer. This argument applies to almost every aspect of health. Some people argue it is better to spend money on prevention than having to spend money on curing diseases that could be prevented. These are the arguments that the Victorians were having (see page 84) when Chadwick and Southwood Smith were saying much the same thing.

Hackney, in London, has adopted a different approach to prevention. It has set up the Healthier Hackney fund. Local communities and voluntary organisations can ask for grants to implement their own attempts to be healthier and to tackle health issues that are important to them. The fund was developed as a new approach for Hackney Council to work with the voluntary and community sector, and a new way to commission health services. The programme is based on the principle that organisations based in the heart of the community have strong connections to residents, know the issues, and often have fresh ideas for unique projects to deal with challenging health issues.

THINK
1. How easy is it to live a healthier lifestyle?
2. Should money be spent on the prevention of disease rather than curing it?

ACTIVITIES
1. How is the Healthier Hackney Fund similar to other attempts at prevention mentioned in this section? How is it different?
2. Which, in your opinion, is more likely to be effective? Why?
3. Conduct some research to see if your local area has any schemes similar to Healthier Hackney

Fitness drives

In August 2009 the health secretary said, 'Promoting active lifestyles is the simple answer to many of the big challenges facing our country today. It can save us money and ease the burden on public services. The NHS has the green light to be bold and creative to help people to be fitter and more healthy.' 'Walking for health' (www.nhs.uk/Livewell/getting-started-guides/Pages/getting-started-walking.aspx) is typical of many fitness drives. It is a campaign designed to encourage people to take more exercise, to walk 10,000 steps a day, at moderate to fast pace. It provides support to gradually build up from no exercise to sufficient exercise. You can access cheap or free swimming classes and get reduced gym membership. 'Be Active' is Birmingham City Council's scheme to provide free leisure services to its residents. Participants register and are given a card which allows them to use a range of facilities from swimming pools and gyms to exercise classes and badminton courts for free during certain times. One-third of the local population has got involved since the project was launched in 2008. Research showed that three-quarters of users were not previously members of a leisure centre, gym or swimming pool and one-half were overweight or obese. It also had a knock-on effect in other areas with rises seen in the numbers seeking help over smoking and alcohol. Overall, for every £1 spent on the scheme £23 is estimated to have been recouped in health benefits.

Healthy eating

'Five-a-day' is perhaps the best known of all the government's health messages. The 'Five-A-Day' campaign is an attempt to get people to eat more fruit and vegetables (see Source L). It has been proven that eating more fruit and vegetables reduces your risk of heart disease and cancer.

The Eatwell Guide, issued in March 2016, is typical of national government campaigns. It depicts a healthy, balanced diet, which includes:

- eating at least five portions of a variety of fruit and vegetables every day
- basing meals on potatoes, bread, rice, pasta or other starchy carbohydrates, ideally wholegrain
- having some dairy or dairy alternatives (such as soya drinks), choosing lower fat and lower sugar options
- eating some beans, pulses, fish, eggs, meat and other proteins (including two portions of fish every week, one of which should be oily)
- choosing unsaturated oils and spreads and consuming in small amounts
- drinking six to eight cups or glasses of fluid a day
- if consuming foods and drinks high in fat, salt and sugar then have these less often and in small amounts.

> **THINK**
> Does this 'Eatwell' guide:
> a) explain clearly the benefits of healthy eating; and
> b) persuade you enough to change any unhealthy habits you might have?

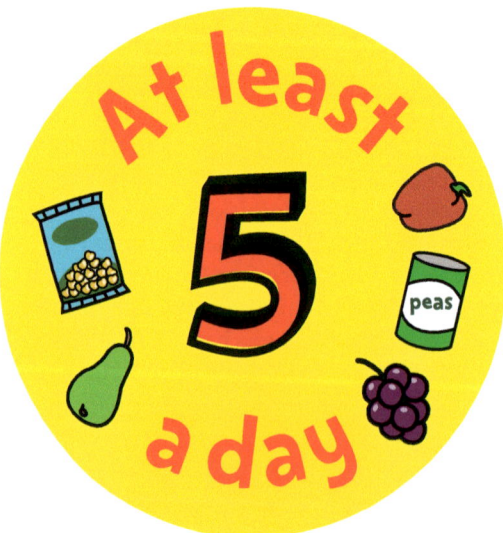

▲ **Source L:** Campaign logo, to encourage us to eat more fruit and vegetables

6 Developments in public health and welfare

FOCUS TASK REVISITED

1. At the beginning of this chapter, you were asked to create tables based on the actions and arguments of the nineteenth-century Clean and Dirty Parties. You will have worked through each section and made lists of actions that might have been, or were, proposed by the Clean Party and the Dirty Party and why they were proposed.
2. Prioritise each list, with the best arguments at the top.
3. Which of the two have, in your opinion, the best arguments? Why?
4. How have the arguments of the Clean Party and the Dirty Party changed over time?
5. Finally, return to the main question we started this chapter with – how effective have attempts been to improve public health and welfare over time? How are you going to measure 'effective'?

ACTIVITIES

1. In pairs, we would like you to produce a worksheet, with the heading, 'Improving public health and welfare.' The target audience is other students studying this course in the future.
2. You might like to consider these ideas:
   a) Why was public health and welfare an issue?
   b) When was the best time to live in towns and cities?
   c) When was the worst time to live in towns and cities?
   d) Whose job was it to improve conditions in towns and cities?
   e) How effective were attempts from the medieval period to today, to improve towns and cities?

Of course, these are only suggestions. It is entirely up to you how you devise your worksheet and what activities you ask other students to do. Have fun!

TOPIC SUMMARY

- In the medieval period towns were more unhealthy than rural areas – but sometimes made strong efforts to improve public health.
- Medieval attempts to clean up towns were not always successful.
- In the seventeenth century towns were healthier than ever.
- The Industrial Revolution completely changed things for the worse, and the government's belief in *laissez-faire* did not help.
- People seemed to split into the Clean Party and the Dirty Party.
- Some individuals worked hard to improve public health in the nineteenth century.
- In the twentieth century government made great efforts to improve public health.
- Many 'new towns' have been set up in an attempt to improve living conditions.
- Now, more emphasis is placed on prevention rather than cure. In particular, lots of emphasis is on healthy living.

Practice questions

1. Describe the methods the mayor and council of Coventry used to try and clean up the town in the fifteenth century. *(For guidance, see page 125.)*
2. Explain why people were unable to effectively clean up towns and cities in the sixteenth and seventeenth centuries. *(For guidance, see page 126.)*
3. Explain why it would be so difficult to improve public health in the new industrial cities of the nineteenth century. *(For guidance, see page 126.)*
4. Outline how attempts to improve public health changed from c.500 to the present day. *(For guidance, see page 127.)*
5. Explain why attempts to improve public health were successful from the early nineteenth century to the end of the twentieth century. *(For guidance, see page 126.)*
6. Look at the three sources:
   - Source A: A modern picture of a medieval town (page 80)
   - Source E: housing in Glasgow in 1868 (page 83)
   - Source K: Cumbernauld new town (page 90)
   Identify one similarity and one difference in public health over time. *(For guidance, see page 121.)*

7 Study of a historic environment: the village of Eyam during the Great Plague of 1665–66

In the autumn of 1665 the 'Great Plague' which was then ravaging the population of London first appeared in the small village of Eyam in Derbyshire with devastating consequences. During the course of the following year over one-third of the population of Eyam died and, in some instances, whole families were wiped out. Yet the plague did not break out in neighbouring towns and villages. The people of Eyam took the selfless action of shutting themselves off from their neighbours and they self-imposed a quarantine zone around their village. In doing so they sacrificed many of the lives of the inhabitants of Eyam for the greater good and their actions stopped the spread of the disease. In this unit you will be investigating how Eyam became an important lesson in the understanding of actions that could be taken to limit the spread of a highly contagious disease and the consequences this had in terms of understanding the control of disease.

FOCUS TASK

As you work through this chapter gather together information to enable you to complete three separate spider diagrams to answer the following questions:
1 What were the key features of the plague?
2 What methods were used to try to limit the spread of the plague?
3 How effective were these methods at limiting the spread of disease?

Plague: the historical context

Plague was a common disease during the medieval and early modern period. It was a disease that had no known cure and caused a high incidence of death among those who contracted the disease.

What was the plague?

There were two types of plague and each was spread in different ways.

Bubonic plague

This was spread by fleas from black rats. When a person was infected by being bitten by a flea carrying the plague bacilli germ, large swellings called buboes appeared in the armpits and the groin. This was followed by a high fever and severe headache, and soon afterwards by the appearance of boils all over the body. Death occurred within a few days. The disease was more common during warmer weather when rats were more numerous and active.

Pneumonic plague

This was spread by people breathing or coughing germs onto one another. The disease attacked the lungs, causing breathing problems. It caused people to cough up blood and death usually occurred quite quickly. Of the two types of plague this tended to be the more dangerous, since it could be spread by direct human contact.

▲ **Source A:** A medieval depiction of the bubonic plague

7 Study of a historic environment: the village of Eyam during the Great Plague of 1665–66

Outbreaks of plague during the medieval period

One of the most devastating pandemic episodes of the bubonic plague was the Black Death which ravaged Europe between 1346 and 1353. This outbreak had its origins on the plains of Central Asia and from there travelled along the Silk Road into the Mediterranean and then on into central and eventually northern Europe (see Figure 7.1). Britain experienced the full force of the Black Death between 1348 and 1349 when between one third and two thirds of the population perished.

Further outbreaks of the plague continued to affect England and Wales for the next three hundred years. Quite severe outbreaks occurred during the years 1361-62, 1369, 1379-83 and 1389-93, with an outbreak in 1471 killing between 10 and 20 per cent of the population. An outbreak in 1479–80 was even more severe, killing an estimated 20 per cent of the population.

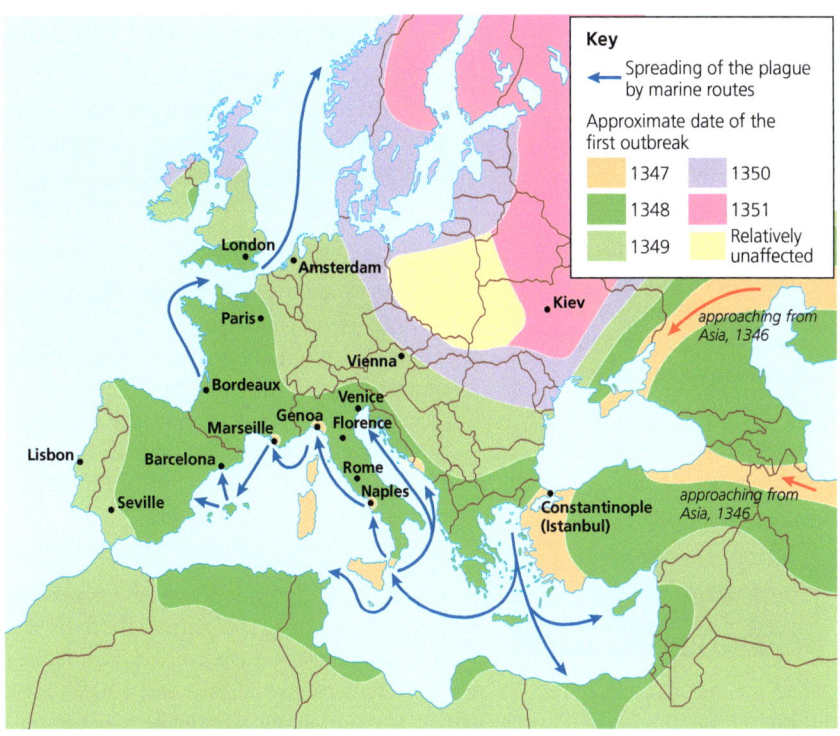

▲ Figure 7.1: Map showing the movement of the Black Death, or plague, into and through Europe

Outbreaks of plague during the sixteenth and seventeenth centuries

The sixteenth century did not escape the disease, with outbreaks being recorded in the years 1535, 1543, 1563 and 1589.

The seventeenth century witnessed further outbreaks in 1603, 1625 and 1636. London was badly affected, recording 30,000 deaths in 1603, 35,000 in 1625 and 10,000 in 1636. The last major epidemic of the plague to occur in England was in 1665-66. It killed over 100,000 people and reduced London's population by over one-quarter. The cause of the deadly disease was the 'Yersinia pestis bacterium' which was transmitted through the bite of an infected rat flea. The fleas lived on the fur of black rats (see Sources B and C).

> **THINK**
>
> 1. Why did people living in medieval times fear the plague?
> 2. 'Pneumonic plague was considered to be a more dangerous form of disease than bubonic plague.' What evidence can you find to support this statement?

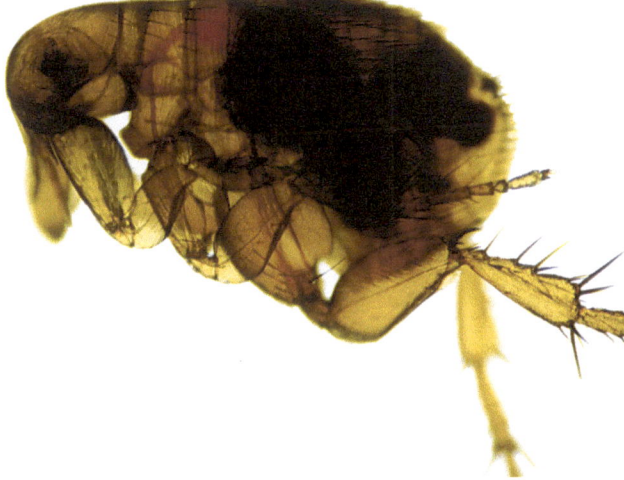

▲ Source B: An image of an infected rat flea. The Yersinia pestis bacteria appears as a dark mass in the gut of the flea. When the flea feeds by biting into the skin of a rat it injects the Yersinia into the wound.

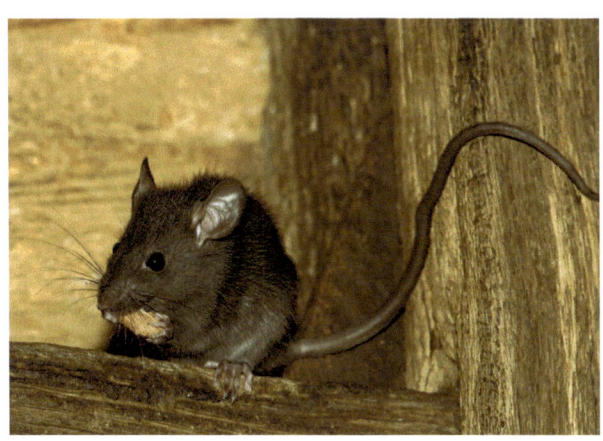

▲ Source C: *Rattus rattus* or the Black Rat, the carrier of the plague

The Great Plague in London, 1665

London was the largest centre of population in the country and plague deaths first began to be reported in the city in April and May of 1665. By July the plague was rampant across the city. Many who had means, including King Charles II and his family, fled the capital to their estates in the countryside. For the poor people, however, there was no option but to stay and face the full force of the epidemic.

The efforts of the authorities to try and contain the epidemic failed.

- Orders were issued to restrict the movement of people in and out of the capital but it was difficult to enforce.
- Theatres and other public entertainments were closed to avoid large gatherings of people.
- Any house containing a plague sufferer had to be sealed up for 40 days and the door marked with a red cross and the words 'Lord have mercy upon us'.
- Dogs and cats were ordered to be caught and killed as it was thought they were carriers of the disease.
- All bodies were to be buried after dark in an attempt to reduce the spread of the disease.

However, this did little to stop the spread of the plague and during the hot weeks of the summer months thousands died. By the end of 1665 the worst was over but the total number of people who had died from the plague in London has been estimated at somewhere between 70,000 and 100,000. By chance, it was the Great Fire of 1666 that helped to cleanse the city of the disease.

> **Source D:** The nursery rhyme *Ring-a-Ring o' Roses* is thought to date back to the time of the Great Plague of 1665–66. The rosy rash was the first sign a person was infected, posies of herbs were thought to offer protection, while sneezing was a final sign that death was close
>
> *Ring-a-ring o' roses,*
> *A pocket full of posies,*
> *A-tishoo! A-tishoo!*
> *We all fall down*

Month	Number of deaths
May	43
June	590
July	4,127
August	19,046
September	26,219
October	14,373
November	3,451
December	940

▲ Table 7.1: Number of deaths from the plague in London during 1665

> **Source E:** Extracts from the diary of Samuel Pepys, a government official who chose not to leave the city during the summer of 1665
>
> *7th June* – This day I did in Drury Lane see two or three houses marked with a red cross upon the doors and 'Lord Have Mercy Upon Us' written there. This worried me so much that I bought a roll of tobacco to smell and chew.
>
> *12th July* – So many are dying that they have to bury some in daylight. [There was not time to bury them all at night.]
>
> *20th July* – There were 1089 dying of the plague this week.
>
> *31st August* – 6102 died of the plague this week. But it is feared that the true number is over 10,000, partly from the poor that cannot be taken notice of.
>
> *15th September* – What a sad time it is! So many people have left London that there are no boats on the river, and grass is growing in Whitehall court.
>
> *26th October* – The town is beginning to be lively again, though the streets are still empty, and most of the shops are shut.

> **THINK**
>
> 1. How useful is Source E to a historian studying the impact of the Great Plague of 1665 upon London?
> 2. Working in pairs, examine the methods used by the authorities in London to try to contain the spread of the disease.
>   a) Do you think Table 7.1 suggests the methods were successful?
>   b) Can you think of reasons why it was difficult to contain the spread of the disease?

Beliefs about the causes

Nobody at this time understood the cause of the Great Plague and there were numerous theories.

- It was sent by God as a punishment for being sinful. People sought divine forgiveness through prayer and by repenting their sins in the hope this would spare them from catching the plague.
- It was caused by bad air which was often referred to as 'miasma'.
- It was spread by cats and dogs.

Medical treatment

Medical treatment was quite primitive and tended to rely upon herbal remedies, nostrums and charms.

- Some carried sweet-smelling flowers to counteract the bad-smelling air or they carried pomanders stuffed with herbs and spices.
- Some men preferred to smoke a pipe of tobacco believing the smoke would kill off the plague; Samuel Pepys bought tobacco to smell and chew in the hope it would protect him against the plague.
- Some believed that bad air spread the infection. Windows and doors were closed and rosemary and incense were burned in the belief it would fumigate the room. In London Samuel Pepys recorded attempts to clear the air by burning coal in braziers placed at intervals along the main streets.
- For those who were infected, poultices were commonly used to draw the lump or bubo to a head, in the belief that when it burst the infection would be drawn off.
- Some took possets, a mixture of boiled milk, ale and bread.

> **Source F:** In his book *Journal of the Plague Year* (1722), the contemporary author Daniel Defoe advised draining the plague from the victim by cutting open or burning the buboes
>
> *The Pain of the Swelling was in particular very violent, and to some intolerable; the Physicians and Surgeons may be said to have tortured many poor Creatures, even to Death.*

The Great Plague was by no means confined to London as trading links and flight caused it to spread to other urban and rural areas. These included the larger settlements of Newcastle and Southampton, as well as small villages such as Eyam.

> **THINK**
> 1. Study Sources F and G. What do they tell you about the methods used to prevent and treat the plague?
> 2. How effective were the methods used by people living in London in 1665 in reducing their chances of catching the plague?

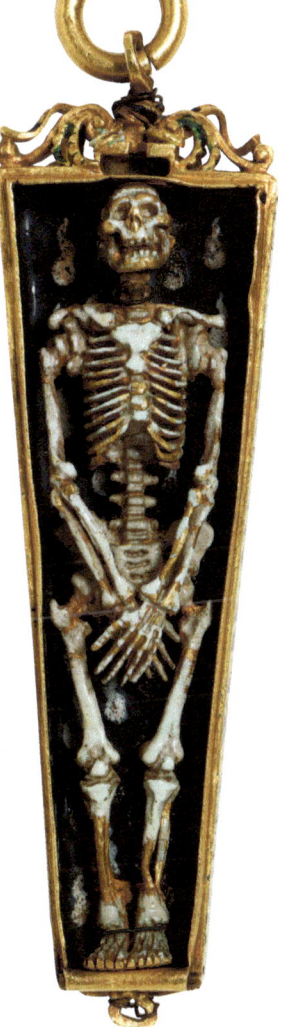
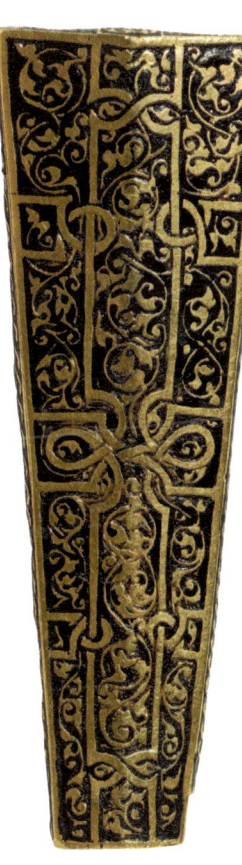

▲ **Source G:** A sixteenth-century pendant. Behind its elegant lid lies a gruesome skeleton, a constant reminder that death could strike anyone, anywhere, at any time. It may also have been intended as a charm to ward off plague

The village of Eyam

Eyam is a small village in Derbyshire which lies between the larger settlements of Buxton and Chesterfield, and just north of Bakewell in the Peak District (see Figure 7.2). Most of the population were farmers who spent their days working the land and tending their animals, or they were employed in the nearby lead mines. In 1665 the population of Eyam stood at around 800 people.

August 1665: the arrival of the plague

It is thought that the plague first reached Eyam in late August 1665 through the arrival of a parcel of cloth sent from London to the village tailor, Alexander Hadfield. Upon opening the parcel the tailors assistant, George Viccars, found the cloth to be damp so he opened it up and spread it out near the fire to dry. Unbeknown to Viccars, the cloth was infested with rat fleas which were carrying the deadly bubonic plague. A very short time afterwards Viccars became ill and within five or six days he was dead. The parish registers record his burial on 7 September 1665.

September–October: the exodus of the richer inhabitants as the disease takes hold

Viccars was the first known fatality from the plague in Eyam, but the infection soon spread rapidly and during the following three weeks there were five further deaths from plague recorded in the parish register:

22 September – young Edward Cooper was buried
23 September – burial of Peter Hawksworth
26 September – burial of Thomas Thorpe
30 September – burial of Mary, 12-year-old daughter of Thomas Thorpe
30 September – burial of Sarah Syddall

During October there were 23 deaths, bringing the total up to 29 by the end of the month. This number of deaths in just two months was more than the average annual number of deaths in the parish of Eyam over the previous decade.

As panic began to set in, those who could afford to shut up their homes and fled the village. About 50 individuals left, among them the Sheldons, a gentry family.

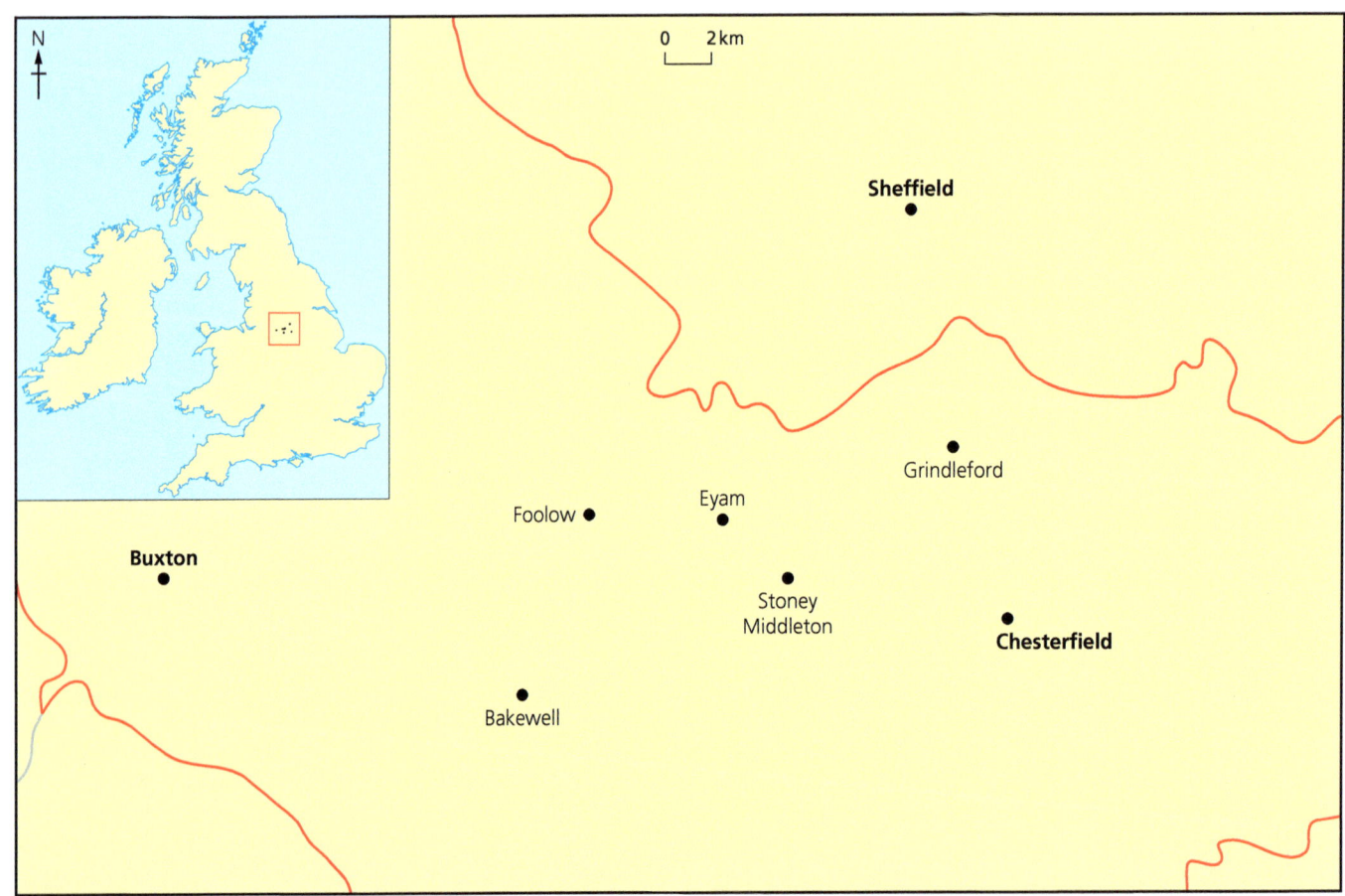

▲ Figure 7.2: A map showing the location of the village of Eyam in relation to its neighbouring larger settlements

7 Study of a historic environment: the village of Eyam during the Great Plague of 1665–66

Winter: a lull during the colder months

As the colder weather began to bite, the spread of the disease appeared to slow down. This was a common feature of bubonic plague, as the rat population declined during the winter months, resulting in less contact with humans. However, once the warmer weather returned the following spring and the rat population increased, there was an increase in the number of humans catching the plague. By April 1666 the total number of deaths from the plague stood at 73 and the lull in the death rate during the early months of the year was suddenly overturned by a dramatic increase in plague deaths during June, July and August (see Table 7.2).

Spring: the plague returns with a vengeance

In June the number of deaths rose above 20 for the first time since the previous October. The month of July witnessed 56 deaths, followed by a further 78 in August. The impact of the plague was now at its worst. During September and October the number of deaths began to fall and in November there was only a single plague death recorded.

Source H: The nineteenth-century local historian William Wood described the return of the plague in June 1666 in his book *The History and Antiquities of Eyam* (1842)

At the commencement of June this deadly monster awoke from his short slumber and with desolating steps stalked forth from house to house, breathing on the terror-struck inhabitants the vapour of death. … As June advanced, the pestilence spread from house to house with dreadful rapidity, sparing neither sex nor age, and it was in that month that the plague began to assume so terrible an aspect.

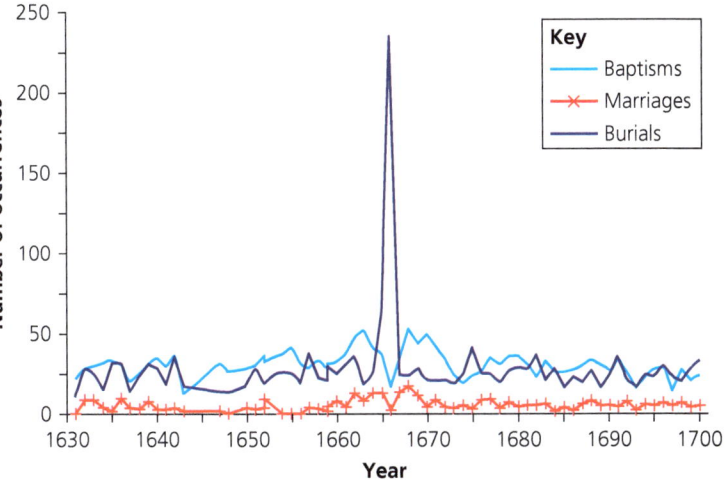

Figure 7.3: A graph showing the number of baptisms, burials and marriages in the parish of Eyam between 1631 and 1700. The information has been obtained from the Eyam Parish Registers

THINK

1 Study Table 7.2. Can you suggest why there was a reduction in the number of deaths from the plague during the winter months, and a dramatic increase during the summer months?
2 Use Source H and your own knowledge to describe the impact of the plague upon the village of Eyam during the summer of 1666.
3 Work in pairs. What information can you extract from Figure 7.3 about the number of baptisms, burials and marriages in the parish of Eyam between 1631 and 1700?

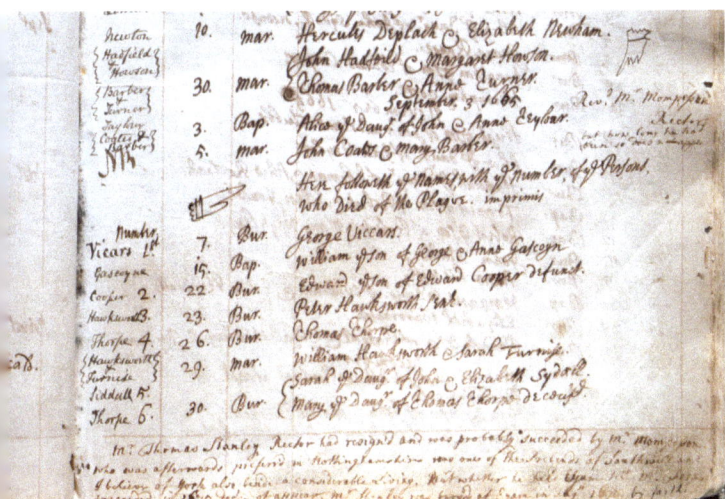

Source I: Parish church records for 1665, citing the first plague mortalities in Eyam

1665 September	6
October	23
November	5
December	8
1666 January	4
February	5
March	2
April	7
May	2
June	21
July	56
August	78
September	24
October	18
November	1
Total number of deaths	260

▲ Table 7.2: Number of plague deaths at Eyam

New methods to combat the plague at Eyam

What is unique about events in Eyam is that the villagers themselves took decisive steps to try to prevent the spread of the disease beyond the immediate village and its neighbouring farms.

The leadership of Mompesson and Stanley

The most important figure in Eyam was its rector, the Rev William Mompesson who lived in the rectory with his wife, Catherine and their two small children. This 28-year-old Oxford-educated rector had only been in his post at the village for a year. However, also still in the village was his predecessor, the Rev Thomas Stanley, a Puritan clergyman who had been dismissed from his post for refusing to take the Oath of Conformity and for refusing to use the new Book of Common Prayer that had been introduced in 1660 upon the restoration of Charles II. Both Mompesson and Stanley were to play important roles in the events of the plague.

It would seem that it was the actions of Mompesson and Stanley that resulted in the setting up of a quarantine zone in order to confine the disease to Eyam and stop it spreading to neighbouring towns, villages and farms. At a distance of half a mile (about 800 m) from the centre of Eyam, a circular boundary was set up all around the village. Villagers were banned from going beyond this line and notices were erected to warn travellers not to enter the quarantine zone which was marked along the key routes by boundary stones. During the whole time the isolation was in force there were almost no attempts to break the quarantine line, even as the infection peaked during the summer of 1666.

Some of the villagers had considered leaving the village for the nearby city of Sheffield but Mompesson persuaded them not to do this as he feared they would spread the plague into the north of England that had more or less escaped the worst of it. In fact, the village decided to cut itself off from the outside world and their sacrifice, which could cost many lives, may well have saved cities in northern England from the worst of the plague.

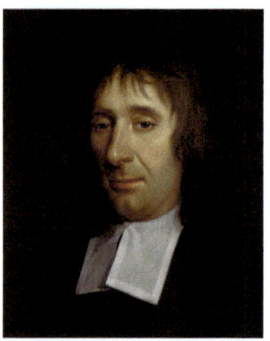

▲ **Source J:** A portrait of the Rev William Mompesson who played a key role in setting up the quarantine zone around Eyam

The quarantine of the village

In setting up a quarantine zone, Mompesson and Stanley gained the acceptance from villagers of a three-point plan.

1. All plague victims were to be buried as quickly as possible and near to their homes rather than in the consecrated ground of the village cemetery. It was correctly thought that this would reduce the risk of the disease spreading from corpses awaiting a burial in the cemetery.
2. They agreed that the church should be locked until the epidemic was over and that all religious services were to be held in the open-air to avoid the risk of the disease spreading among parishioners crammed together in pews. The open air services were held in a small valley known as the Delph and Mompesson preached standing on top of a rock called 'Cucklett Church'.
3. The establishment of a cordon sanitaire around the village beyond which no Eyam resident could pass. This seemed to be the only effective means of controlling the extent of the outbreak.

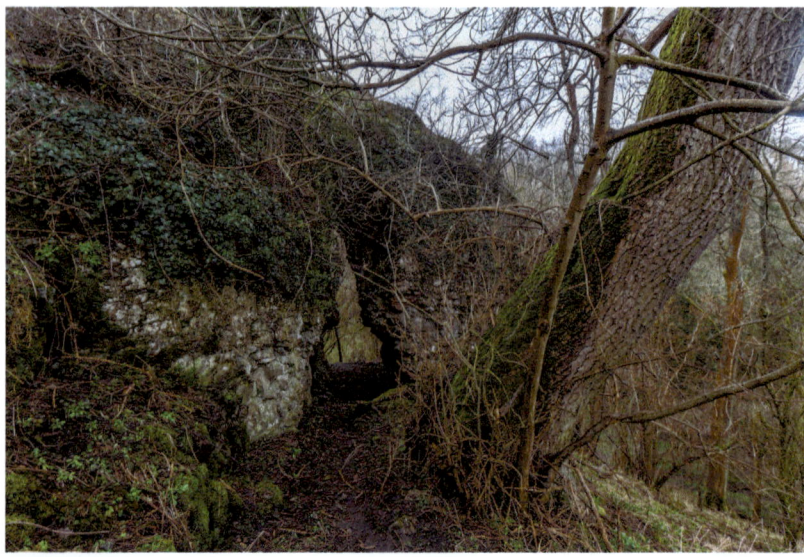

▲ **Source K:** Cucklett Church

7 Study of a historic environment: the village of Eyam during the Great Plague of 1665–66

However, the village of Eyam was not self-supporting. To ensure that villagers did not starve to death they were supplied with food and other essentials from surrounding villages. The Earl of Devonshire, who lived at nearby Chatsworth House, together with some other wealthy neighbours provided supplies which were left at the southern boundary of the village. The boundary stones served as dropping-off points for supplies of food, medicine and other goods. There were several dropping-off points, supplies from Foolow being left at Mompesson's well, a mile from the centre of the village. To pay for the supplies the villagers left money in water troughs filled with vinegar. It was thought that vinegar would kill off the disease.

These measures helped to ensure that the disease did not spread beyond Eyam to the neighbouring villages of Bakewell, Fulwood and beyond.

An area of dispute between historians concerns whether it was Mompesson or Stanley who played the more dominant and decisive role in organising and enforcing the quarantine, as the following Sources M and N illustrate.

> **Source M:** Writing in his book *Spiritualibus Pecci* (1702) the Puritan minister, William Bagshaw, implied that Mompesson played no part in the decision to isolate the village
>
> *It was more reasonable, that the whole Country should in more than Words testifie their Thankfulness to him [Stanley], who together with his Care of the Town, had taken such Care, as no one else did, to prevent the Infection of the Towns adjacent.*

> **THINK**
>
> 1 Study the three-point plan for the introduction of a quarantine zone. Which of the three measures was:
>   a) most effective in stopping the spread of the plague beyond Eyam, and
>   b) most effective in limiting the spread of the disease within the village of Eyam itself?
>
> 2 Why do Sources M and N have different views about whether it was Mompesson or Stanley who played the most important role in organising the quarantine zone?

> **Source N:** An extract taken from an article about the plague at Eyam which was written by William Seward, a supporter of the established Church, in an article published in the *European Magazine* (1793)
>
> *England may congratulate herself in having cherished in her bosom a Parish Priest [Mompesson], who, without the splendour of character, ... watched over the flock committed to his charge at no less risqué of life, and with not less fervour of piety and activity of benevolence.*

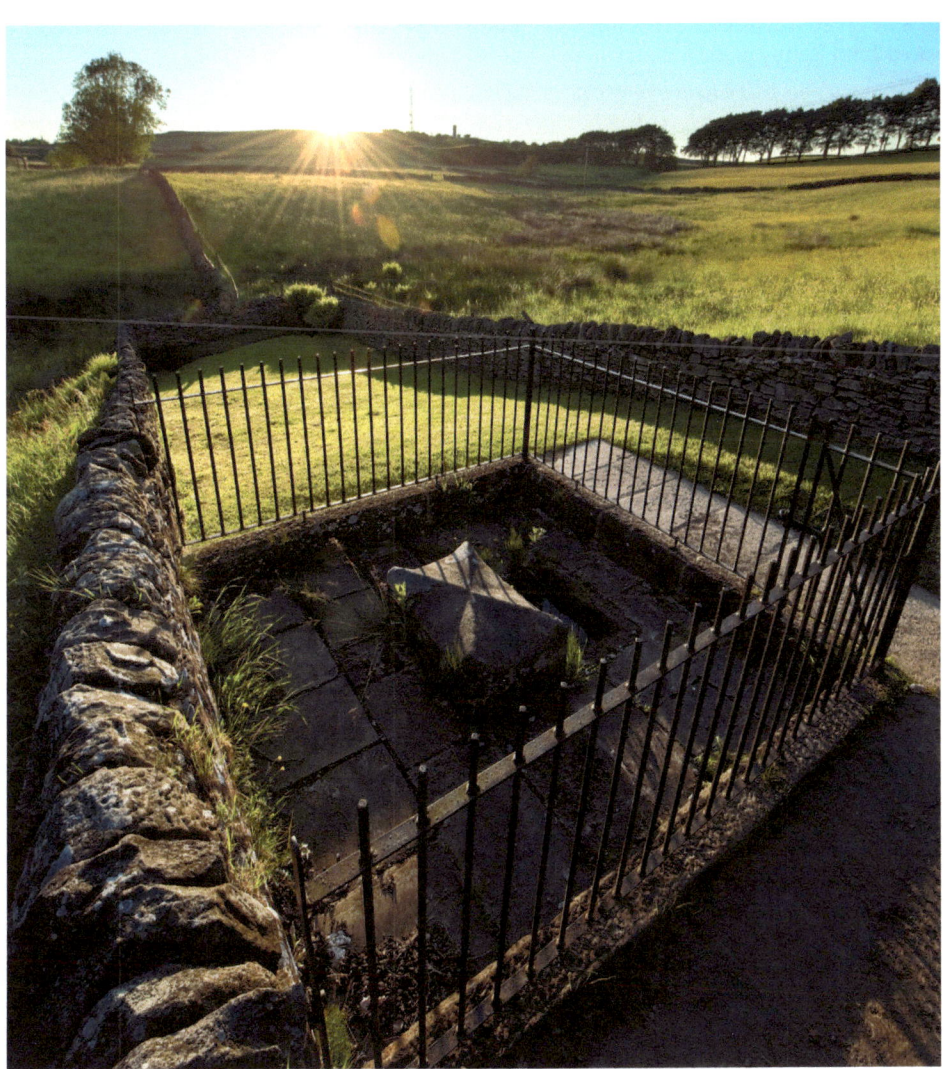

◀ **Source L:** Mompesson's Well which marked the start of the quarantine zone. It was one of the dropping off points for supplies from Foolow

The consequences of the Great Plague visiting Eyam

By choosing to isolate itself the village of Eyam paid a heavy price from the visitation of the Great Plague. Had villagers been allowed to leave, their lives may well have been saved, but in leaving they ran a greater risk of spreading the disease to neighbouring settlements, a risk they chose to avoid.

The human cost of the tragedy

The plague ended in Eyam in October 1666. Over a 14-month period it had claimed the lives of 260 inhabitants, out of an original population of about 800. While there has been some dispute among historians as to the actual size of Eyam's population just prior to the plague, with figures ranging from between 350 and 800, recent calculations based upon Eyam's Hearth Tax returns confirm a figure of just under 800 souls. Whatever the figure, what is clear is that the percentage of the population of Eyam that died was exceptionally high and exceeded the percentage of those who died of Plague in London in 1665 (17 per cent). According to Mompesson, 76 families were affected by the plague, some paying a very heavy price. At the farm of Riley, on the outskirts of the village, Mrs Elizabeth Hancock buried her husband and six children in a space of just eight days.

> **Source O:** On 20 November 1666, once the plague was over, the Rev William Mompesson wrote to John Beilby of York describing what he had experienced at Eyam
>
> *The condition of this place hath been so dreadful that I persuade myself it exceedeth all history and example. I may truly say our Town has become a Golgotha, a place of skulls. ... My ears never heard such doleful lamentations. My nose never smelt such noisome smells, and my eyes never beheld such ghastly spectacles. Here have been 76 families visited within my parish, out of which died 259 persons.*

> **THINK**
>
> How useful are Sources O and P to historians studying the impact of the plague upon the village of Eyam?

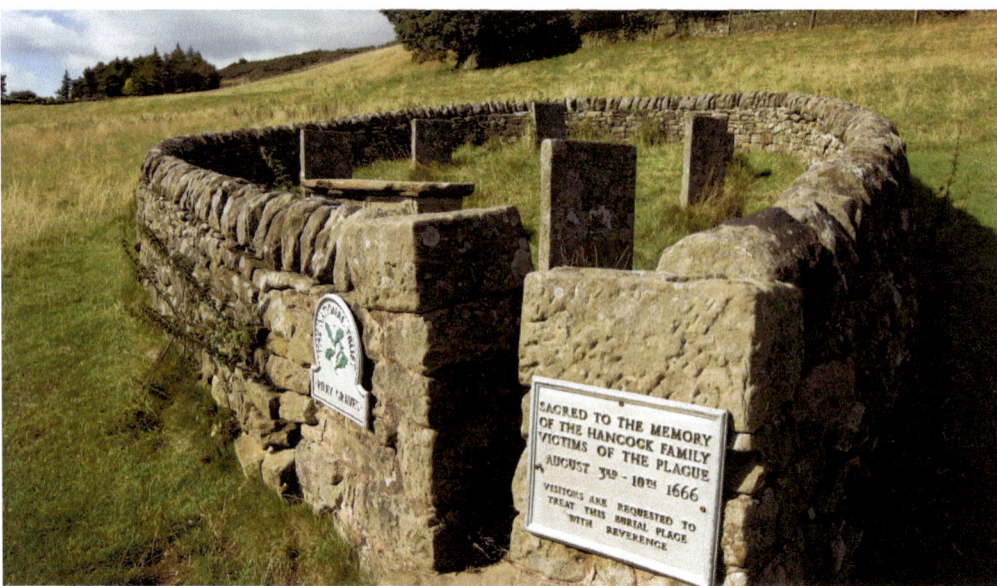

▲ **Source P:** Photograph showing the preserved remains of the Riley graves as they appear today

7 Study of a historic environment: the village of Eyam during the Great Plague of 1665–66

Case studies

The deaths recorded in the Eyam Parish Registers reveal the heavy price paid by many families in both the village of Eyam itself and its neighbouring farms.

The human cost at Eyam

The Hawksworth family
The head of the family was Peter who lived with his wife Jane and their 18-month-old son, Humphrey. Jane was also pregnant with their second child. Peter was the third victim of the plague, followed shortly after by the death of Jane's mother. Next to perish was Jane's brother and his wife, followed by young Humphrey, just three weeks after his father. Over the following months Jane lost 25 members of her extended family. To add to this tragedy, when her baby was born in March 1666 it died within a couple of days, but not from the plague. Jane was now alone and her world had been turned upside down.

The Mompesson family
William sent his two young children away to Sheffield in June 1666 and he wanted his wife to go with them. Catherine however wished to stay to help her husband tend the dying and give comfort to those who had lost family members. Catherine contracted the disease and when she died on 25 August she became the 200th person in the village to die from the plague. William Mompesson remarried in 1670, obtained a new church post and moved to the parish of Eakring in Nottinghamshire. He was to live at Eakring for a further 38 years before he died in 1708.

The Thorpe family
There were nine people living in the Thorpe house, all of them died as a result of catching the plague. William Thorpe left a will but none of his immediate family survived to inherit and his legacy was eventually split between distant relatives living in neighbouring villages.

The Morten family
The Morten family were farmers who lived on the edge of the village. When Mrs Morten was in labour with her third child nobody would come to the house to help with the delivery as one of her other children was dying of the plague. The disease spread through the house and Mrs Morten and all her three children died (boy aged three, girl aged two and the baby just born). They were buried by Mr Morten close to their home. Only Mr Morten survived.

The Talbot family
All of the Talbot family perished as a result of the plague. Richard Talbot was the village blacksmith and he was the first Talbot to die in early July. He was soon followed by Mary (aged 30), his wife, and Mary (aged 18), his daughter, both of whom were buried on 5 July. Mary's sisters, Anne (aged 6) and Jane (aged 8) died on the 7 and 17 July. Six more family members had died by the end of the month and on 15 August, 'old Mrs Bridget Talbot' died. The last to die was Catherine, Bridget's great grandchild, a baby just three months old. There was only one survivor of the Talbot family, George, the eldest son who was working away from the village. He eventually returned to Eyam and took over the smithy which had been run by his father.

The Blackwell family
Margaret Blackwell was the sole survivor of this family, her children and husband having perished during the early part of 1666. Margaret caught the disease and appeared to be in the late stages of suffering when she pulled through and went on to live a long life.

The Hancock family
The Hancocks were the neighbours of the Talbots. The first of the Hancocks to die was a child on 3 August. By the 10 August Mr Hancock and his five remaining children had all died. Only Mrs Hancock survived. She later left the village and went to live with her one remaining son who worked in Sheffield.

▲ Figure 7.4: The cost to families in Eyam

> **THINK**
> Can you think of reasons why families like the Hawksworths and the Talbots were so badly affected by the plague?

103

Consequences

By Christmas of 1666 the plague had died out and life was slowly beginning to return to normal, or as normal as it could be for a village which had lost one-third of its inhabitants. The quarantine was lifted and those who had originally fled began to return home. In an attempt to prevent further outbreaks of the plague a 'great burning' was organised. Mompesson set the example and proceeded to burn almost everything but the clothes he stood up in. There was a belief that these items held the plague 'seeds' and therefore had to be destroyed.

In reality the quarantine had proved to be effective as there were no deaths outside the parish and nowhere else in Derbyshire was afflicted by the plague. However, the visit of the Great Plague did have a long-term demographic effect.

- The most obvious effect was a sharp fall in population immediately after 1666. This was followed by a sharp rise between 1667–70, probably accounted for by the return of people who had fled the village in 1665–66. After 1670 there was a steady but slow rise in population but by 1700 the figure was still well below what it had been in 1665.
- The mortality rate in Eyam in 1665–66 was extremely high. It had a ratio of epidemic to average burials of 10.2. By comparison the 47 parishes in London during the Great Plague of the same period had a ratio of 5.9, just over one-half that of Eyam.
- The Eyam Parish Registers reveal that the number of baptisms entered a period of sharp decline after 1666, most likely due to the fact that there were few adults of child-bearing age (see Table 7.3).
- It had an immediate impact upon the local economy – farms were left empty, the land was uncultivated until somebody could take it over and key businesses and trades were left unfilled until new people with such trades moved into the village. Some of the vacancies took many years to fill.

> **THINK**
> 1. Identify (a) the immediate and (b) the longer term impact of the visit of the plague to the village of Eyam during 1665–66.
> 2. Use Source Q and your own knowledge to explain the effectiveness of the use of a quarantine zone.

The effectiveness of the quarantine

The decision of the villagers of Eyam to agree to quarantine themselves from neighbouring settlements undoubtedly stopped the disease from spreading. It is a unique example of community action by a few to save the greater number. The Victorian local historian William Wood was in no doubt about the importance of the sacrifice made by the people of Eyam (see Source Q).

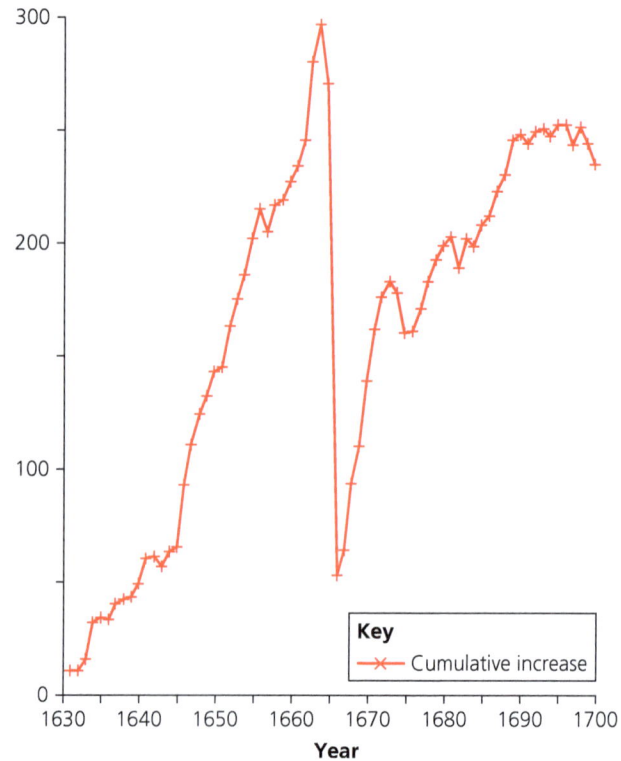

▲ Figure 7.5: A graph showing the population trend based upon figures taken from Eyam Parish Register

Year	Mean annual number of baptisms
1651–60	34.1
1661–70	42.0
1671–80	31.0
1681–90	28.7
1691–1700	24.2

▲ Table 7.3: Number of baptisms in Eyam in the second half of the seventeenth century

> **Source Q:** William Wood, *The History and Antiquities of Eyam*, (1842)
>
> Let all who tread the green fields of Eyam remember, with feelings of awe and veneration, that beneath their feet repose [rest] the ashes of those moral heroes, who with a sublime, heroic and unparalleled resolution gave up their lives, yea doomed themselves to pestilential death to save the surrounding country. ... Their magnanimous [generous] self-sacrifice in confining themselves within a proscribed boundary during the terrible pestilence, is unequalled in the annals of the world. The plague, which would undoubtedly have spread from place to place through the neighbouring counties, was here hemmed in, and in a dreadful and desolating struggle, destroyed and buried with its victims.

The significance of Eyam for changing attitudes towards the prevention of disease

While in the immediate term the events at Eyam did little to directly change attitudes towards the prevention of disease, in the longer term doctors and medical staff were able to reflect upon the significance and consequences of actions taken at Eyam and learn from them.

- Doctors came to realise that the use of a quarantine zone, if actively enforced, could prevent the spread of disease from one infected settlement to neighbouring settlements.
- This is a method commonly used today in the farming world to limit the spread of diseases such as foot and mouth.
- However, it was not until the nineteenth century and the work of Florence Nightingale that patients in hospitals with infectious diseases were isolated in particular wards, thereby adopting the lessons of quarantine pioneered at Eyam. The isolating of wards infected with the norovirus is a modern example of what happened at Eyam.
- Doctors also became aware that methods could be adopted to reduce the risk of contamination. At Eyam this was done by paying for food supplies by dropping coins into pots of vinegar or water, preventing the coins from being directly handed over (see Source R).
- Eyam also attempted to limit the spread of disease by the quick disposal of infected bodies close to the immediate area of death. This limited the risk of spreading the disease, a practice recently adopted in Africa to deal with the Ebola epidemic.
- At Eyam, Mompesson ordered the burning of contaminated items. During the nineteenth century this was taken a stage further through developments in improving hygiene and the sterilisation of equipment and medical clothing.

> **THINK**
>
> Do you think the events at Eyam during the plague years did much to change attitudes towards the prevention of disease?

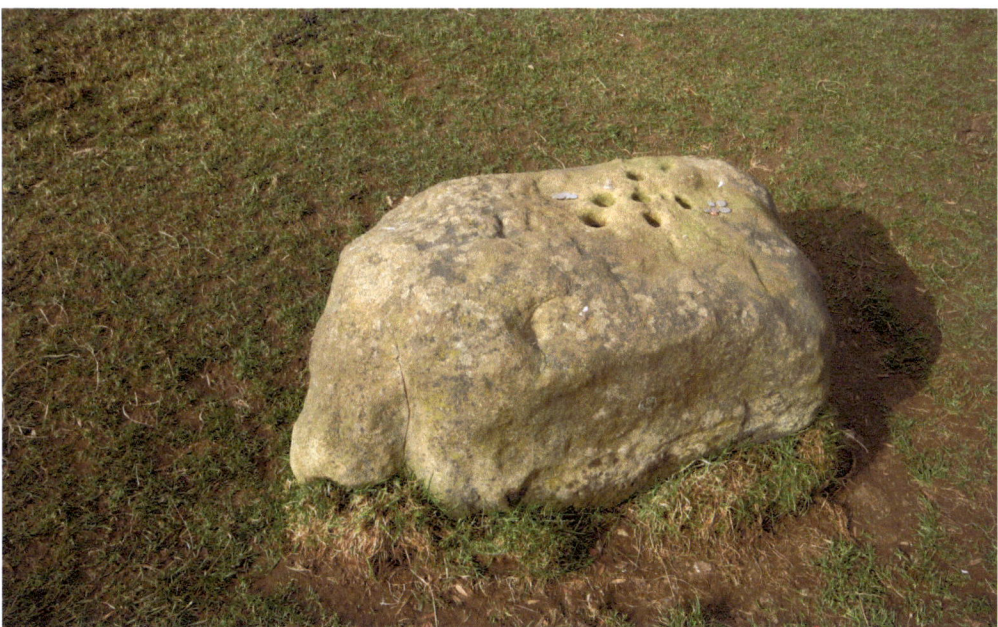

Source R: The boundary stone at Eyam, the plague village in Derbyshire, where coins were left in vinegar to pay for food from neighbours

FOCUS TASK REVISITED

Look back over the three spider diagrams you have constructed as you worked through this chapter. Use your findings to answer the following questions:
1 How successful were the methods used in Eyam to limit the spread of the disease?
2 Were the actions of the inhabitants of Eyam more successful than the actions of the authorities in London in stopping the plague from spreading? Give reasons to support your answer.

ACTIVITIES

Divide into groups of four or five to complete the following task.

In today's world we are told that there is an increasing chance of the emergence of a disease which is resistant to treatment from antibiotics. If such a disease which proved to be highly contagious and had a high rate of death following infection was to break out, what action do you think the government should take to:
1 limit the spread of the disease
2 reduce the high rate of death?

Share and compare the recommendations of the different groups in your class.

TOPIC SUMMARY

- Plague was a deadly disease which resulted in a high death rate.
- There were two types of plague – bubonic and pneumonic.
- England was visited by a severe outbreak of the bubonic plague during 1665–66.
- The disease was spread by fleas living in the fur of black rats.
- London was badly affected and the attempts to limit the spread of the disease within the city had only limited effect.
- Other parts of England were affected by the plague, one of the worst being the village of Eyam in Derbyshire.
- Plague first visited Eyam during the autumn of 1665, with the epidemic dying down during the winter months.
- The spring of 1666 saw a resurgence of the plague with high numbers of deaths during the summer months.
- The rector William Mompesson and Thomas Stanley, the former rector, took decisive action to prevent the disease from spreading by persuading the villagers to set up a quarantine zone around Eyam.
- Neighbouring villages supplied food and other materials, leaving the items at the boundary stones set up at the edge of the quarantine zone.
- The inhabitants of Eyam paid a heavy price for their isolation and some families were wiped out completely.
- However, the quarantine zone prevented the plague from spreading to other parts of Derbyshire.
- Eyam provides an example of how isolation of an infection can help to stop the spread of disease.

Practice questions

1 Describe two immediate results of the arrival of the Great Plague in Eyam in 1665.
2 Explain why the environment of Eyam during the Great Plague was significant in influencing the methods used to fight the spread of disease in the seventeenth century.

8 Study of a historic environment: the British sector of the Western Front, 1914–18, and the treatment and care of the wounded

Between 1914 and 1918 British and French forces fought a war against Germany, a war which did not involve the movement of troops across wide areas but the opposite; intense fighting over a small contained piece of land. The generals were forced to adopt new tactics and, in an attempt to gain an advantage, new weapons and new technology were introduced which caused death and injury on a scale not seen in any previous wars. Casualty rates were high, and the types of wounds and injuries sustained by the soldiers forced medical services to develop new methods of caring for and treating the wounded. In this unit you will investigate how the fighting in the British sector of the Western Front contributed to changes in the methods and procedures of treating and caring for the wounded in battle.

FOCUS TASK

As you work through this chapter complete the table below, which requires you to identify the medical advances in the treatment of the wounded and to evaluate the degree of success. One example has been completed for you. Add extra rows as needed.

What problems faced medical staff treating the wounded on the Western Front?	What attempts were made to overcome these problems?	What was the impact of these new developments/methods?
High death rate from thigh bone injuries which got infected.	The invention and widespread adoption of the 'Thomas Splint'.	Reduced the death rate from thigh bone injury from 80% to 20%

Historical content: a new type of warfare

In the late summer of 1914 war broke out in Europe and spread to become a World War. The war lasted four years and did not end until November 1918. It caused death and injury to armed personnel on a scale never seen before in human history.

Conventional warfare

Before 1914 wars had traditionally been wars of movement in which field guns had been used to weaken and tear holes in the enemy lines. This would then allow the infantry soldiers, assisted by the cavalry, to move forward to attack and capture the weakened position, causing the enemy to either surrender of retreat.

Stalemate and trench warfare

The type of warfare that began to emerge in Western Europe by the end of 1914 was the opposite to a war of movement. The fighting had now become bogged down in one spot, with neither side capable of inflicting a knock-out blow against the other. In this situation of stalemate both sides were forced to dig in and oppose each other across a narrow stretch of no-man's land. This new type of conflict became a war of attrition with each side attempting to wear down the other. The conflict developed into a defensive one in which the priority was to kill or wound as many of the enemy as possible and destroy their equipment before they destroyed yours. The name given to this type of conflict was trench warfare.

Planning medical aid

Nobody could have predicted the development of a static war in which trench warfare became the main form of fighting. This type of war was not planned for and it had serious consequences for the medical planning needed to deal with the high incidences of wounds, injuries and illnesses resulting from fighting in such close range. Medical aid had to adapt quickly to this new type of fighting, which involved the treatment of high numbers of casualties; both the immediate treatment of soldiers wounded on the front line, as well as the longer-term care and treatment of wounded soldiers.

The development of trench warfare

The war in Europe was fought on several fronts, one of the most intensive areas of fighting being the Western Front where the Allied forces of Britain, France and Belgium (together with the USA from 1917) faced the Kaiser's army of Imperial Germany. The Western Front stretched from the coast of the English Channel in Belgium to the French border with Switzerland, a distance of around 700 km (see Figure 8.1).

To begin with trenches were dug very quickly and very simply, being only intended as temporary shelter for the troops. However, as the war dragged on and trenches became a more permanent fixture, they became more sophisticated and they developed into a highly effective defensive network.

The trench system

Trenches were very difficult to capture since the trench system consisted of at least three lines of defence. The front-line trench was supported by a support trench and behind that was a reserve trench. They were connected to each other by communication trenches (see Figure 8.2). Trenches were usually zig-zagged so that if the enemy captured a section they could not fire down its length or, if a shell landed in the trench its explosion would be absorbed into the zig-zagged sides rather than blow away all the soldiers right down the trench line.

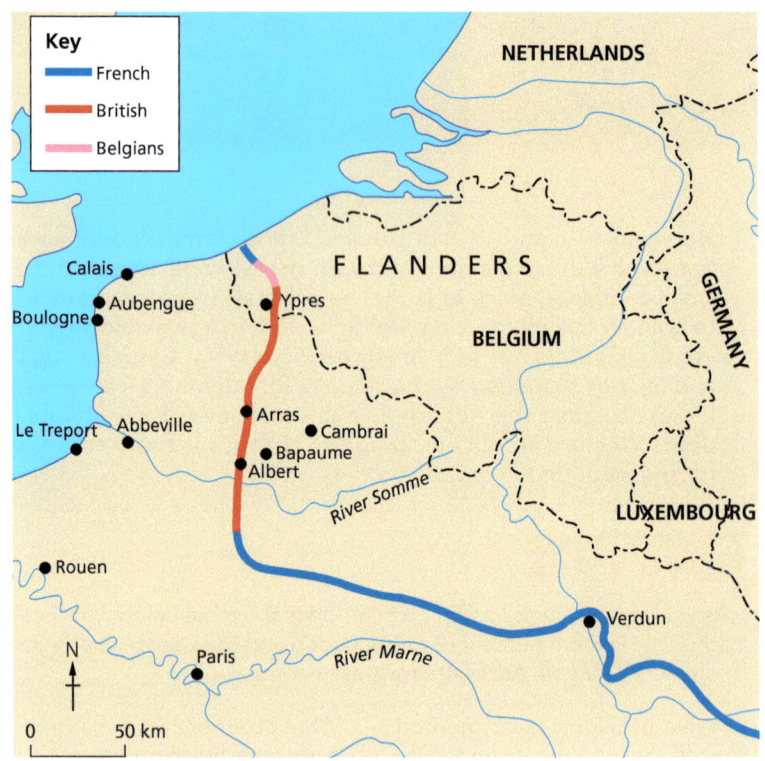

▲ Figure 8.1: The British sector on the Western Front

The features of a trench

A typical trench was several metres deep with sand bags at slightly above head height to protect occupants from sniper fire. A firing step was used by soldiers to peer over the sandbags across no-man's land and within the trench dug-outs were used for shelter during times of shelling or to shelter from bad weather. At regular intervals there would be a machine-gun post and, to slow down movement across no-man's land, coils of barbed wire were laid out by both sides. The big guns of the heavy artillery were situated behind the reserve line of trenches and they were used to bombard the enemy trenches prior to an attack. Such defences made it extremely difficult for the enemy to break through the trench system and any attack would result in high numbers of dead and injured soldiers.

Time at the front

Life at the front was not one of constant fighting. Typically over a 32-day period a soldier would spend:

- eight days in a front-line trench
- eight days in a reserve trench in case of an attack
- 16 days away from the front in the nearest town or village.

However, this would change if an offensive was taking place.

> **THINK**
> 1. How did trench warfare differ from the type of fighting in previous wars?
> 2. 'For soldiers fighting in the trenches the chances of being wounded or killed were very high.' What evidence can you find to support this statement?

8 Study of a historic environment: the British sector of the Western Front, 1914–18

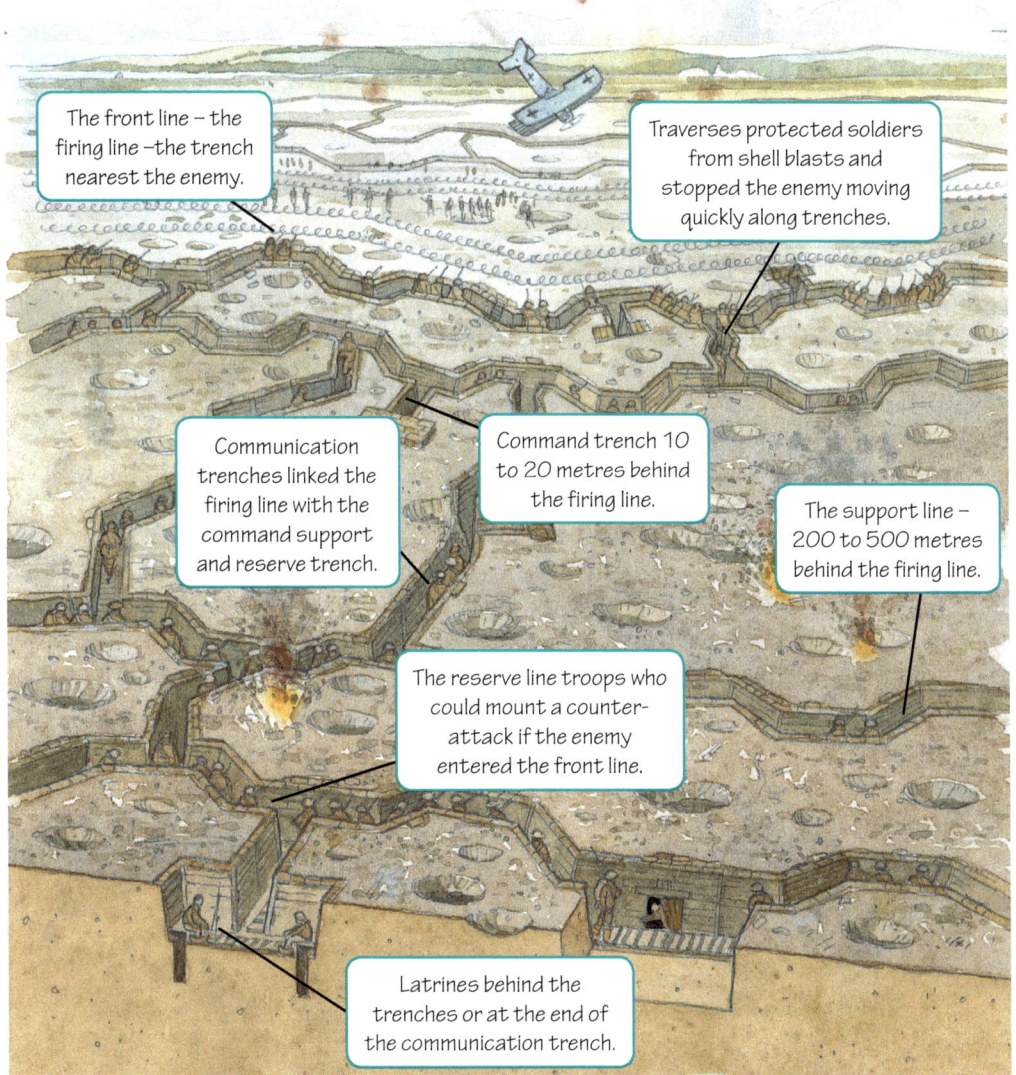

Soldiers spent about 15 per cent of their time in the front line.

Soldiers spent about 10 per cent of their time in the support trench.

Soldiers spent about 30 per cent of their time in the reserve line.

Soldiers spent about 45 per cent of their time away from the trenches.

◄ Figure 8.2: The layout of the trench system

Parapet – A bank of earth thrown up in front of the trench itself to allow a man to fire from the trench with a rest for his elbows and as much protection from incoming fire as possible. Parapets were required to stop a German rifle bullet. They were therefore four- to five-feet thick.

Parados – Was the equivalent of the parapet but behind the trench. It was designed to stop bullets carrying on to the next line of trenches and to shield men from the blast of a shell exploding behind them.

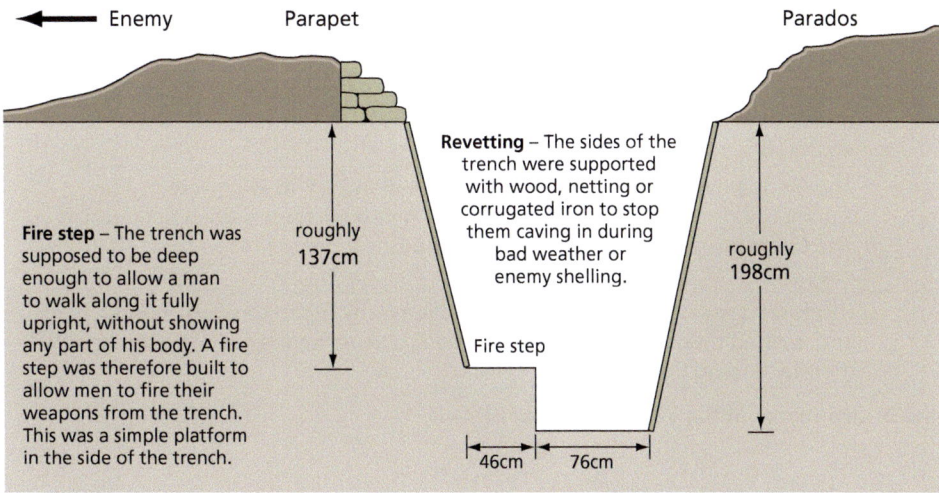

◄ Figure 8.3: A cross-section of a trench

THINK

1 Study Figure 8.2. Explain why the trench system was:
   a) difficult to attack
   b) resulted in high numbers of casualties.

2 Study Figure 8.3. Explain the function of each of the following features found within a trench system:
   a) revetting;
   b) paradus;
   c) sand bags.

109

The nature of trench warfare

The generals who directed British forces along the Western Front have been criticised for repeatedly using tactics which were predictable and which cost the lives of so many. However, the generals believed that in order to break through the stalemate they had to follow a policy of attrition, wearing the enemy down by constant attack. They were convinced that a breakthrough would come if enough troops were concentrated along a small sector of the front, forcing the enemy line to break. What they could not deal with was the fact that the enemy could quickly bring in reserves from other sectors to plug any gaps in their front line. As a result of such conflict casualty figures were extremely high and were accentuated by:

- weapons capable of mass killing – machine guns could mow down charging soldiers
- gas – used for the first time in 1915
- heavy artillery – big, powerful guns could kill and injure hundreds of soldiers during a bombardment
- the problem of crossing no-man's land – barbed wire, lack of cover and shell craters often filled with water – made soldiers easy targets for enemy snipers and machine gunners
- the infantry now replaced the cavalry as the main fighting weapon, until the development of the tank.

Trench warfare re-wrote the rules of warfare and forced a radical re-think in the provision of medical care and treatment of wounded soldiers.

Major offensives along the Western Front

British forces played a major role in defending a line of trenches along the Western Front. They fought a number of key battles, many of which resulted in high casualty figures.

Date	Battle	Description
August–September 1914	Battle of the Marne	This was a turning point as it stopped the German advance. It ended the Schlieffen Plan and resulted in stalemate as both sides began digging themselves in to protect themselves against snipers and shell fire.
October–November 1914	First Battle of Ypres	A German advance was stopped but both sides suffered heavy losses. The result was deadlock.
April–May 1915	Second Battle of Ypres	In a renewed attack the Germans used chlorine gas for the first time and almost achieved a breakthrough but British and Canadian reinforcements saved the situation. Both sides experienced heavy losses and Allied casualties were estimated at 60,000.
July–November 1916	Battle of the Somme	The battle took place between 1 July and 17 November 1916 over a 22-kilometre length of trench system in the Somme region. It was an attempt by the British to force German troops away from Verdun to relieve the pressure on the French army. By the end of the first day 19,240 British soldiers had been killed and there were over 60,000 casualties.
April–May 1917	Battle of Arras	During the spring of 1917 the British and French attacked German positions at Arras but little ground was captured. Casualties were very high.
July–November 1917	Third Battle of Ypres	The British launched a major attack aimed at dislodging the Germans from high ground and capturing Passchendaele Ridge near the town of Ypres. The bloody assault left both sides exhausted and the ground turned to mud because of constant rain. The ridge was captured but at a cost of 245,000 casualties and the death of 47,000 British soldiers.
November–December 1917	Battle of Cambrai	This was the first occasion when the British used tanks massed together to attack German trenches. It failed to break through German lines and resulted in 40,000 British casualties.
Spring 1918	German Offensive	The German army launched a major attack along an 80-kilometre front, aiming to bring the war to an end before American forces arrived in Europe. The Germans failed to break through. The British experienced over 200,000 casualties.
Summer–Autumn 1918		Reinforced with American troops the Allied army broke through German lines and pushed them back. Germany agreed to an armistice on 11 November 1918 thereby ending fighting on the Western Front.

▲ Table 8.1: Key battles fought along the British sector of the Western Front, 1914–18

8 Study of a historic environment: the British sector of the Western Front, 1914–18

> **ACTIVITY**
>
> Study Table 8.1 and Source A.
>
> Working in pairs:
> 1. Identify three reasons why casualty figures were so high in the battles of Ypres, the Somme and Cambrai.
> 2. Rank these reasons in order of importance, explaining the reasons for your choice.
> 3. Share your findings with the rest of the class.

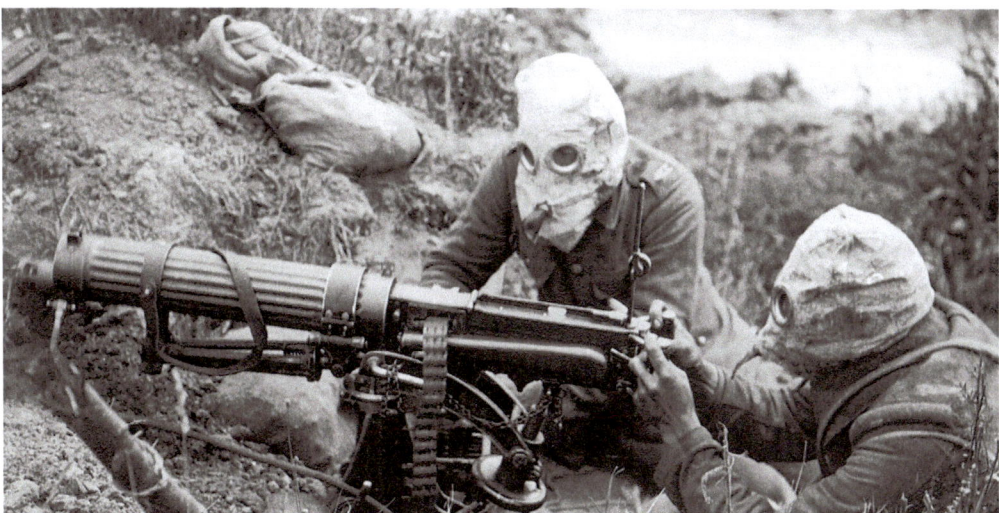

▲ **Source A:** A water-cooled Vickers machine gun crew wearing anti-gas masks in July 1916 during the Battle of the Somme

Wounds and injuries

During the course of the war over 22 million men were wounded, either physically or psychologically. Medical services found themselves facing casualties with severe wounds and injuries received from a variety of weapons.

- Rifles – these were automatic rapid fire guns, which fired bullets with a pointed tip, designed to go deeper into the body from a longer distance.
- Machine guns – these were capable of firing up to 500 rounds per minute and they could have a devastating impact against advancing soldiers attempting to cross no-man's land.
- Artillery – the British developed the Howitzer guns which could fire powerful shells a distance of over 19 km; such shells were the cause of over one-half of all injuries sustained by soldiers at the front.

Rifle, bayonet and machine gun wounds

Bullets fired from rifles and machine guns had the power to break major bones and pierce vital organs such as the liver and kidneys. Over 60,000 British soldiers suffered bullet wounds to the head and eyes, and over 41,000 men had to have limbs amputated due to gunshot wounds. Major injuries could also be inflicted through the use of the bayonet.

Shelling and shrapnel wounds

Artillery shells were the weapon soldiers feared the most and they were the biggest cause of casualties. They were designed to explode 4 or 5 m above the ground, causing maximum casualties. Jagged fragments of the iron casing and hundreds of metal fragments inside them could easily tear off a limb and shatter bones.

Gas attacks

Chlorine gas was first used by the German army in April 1915 during the Second Battle of Ypres and to begin with soldiers had no protection. Three types of gas were used at the front:

- Chlorine gas: this caused immediate choking due to the gas stripping away the linings of the lungs, causing the victims to drown from water produced in their own lungs.
- Phosgene gas: this was 18 times more deadly than chlorine gas although its impact was not immediate and it took the victim 48 hours to die, having experienced spasms and vomiting followed by their lungs filling up with a yellow liquid which caused them to drown.
- Mustard gas: this was first used in 1917 and was not that deadly; only 2 per cent of victims died. However, it did attack the surface of the skin causing intense burning, swelling of the eyes, blindness and choking.

The effects of gas were limited and after 1916, following the introduction of gas masks, only 3 per cent of gassed soldiers died and 93 per cent of men were able to return to duty. What gas attacks did do, however, was to clog up treatment areas with doctors having to give sufferers oxygen and wash the skin thoroughly to remove traces of poison gas.

> **Source B:** An account of the effects of mustard gas recorded by a British nurse, S. Millard, in her book *I Saw Them Die* (1936)
>
> Gas cases are terrible. They cannot breathe lying down or sitting up. They just struggle for breath, but nothing can be done. Their lungs are gone – literally burnt out. Some have their eyes and faces entirely eaten away by gas … One boy today, screaming to die, the entire top layer of his skin, burnt from face and body. I gave him an injection of morphine.

Year	Casualties	Deaths
1915	12,792	307
1916	6,698	1,123
1917	52,452	1,796
1918	113,764	2,673

▲ Table 8.2: Official statistics for casualties and deaths caused by gas in the British army, 1915–18

> **THINK**
>
> Why did many soldiers come to fear artillery shells more than any other weapon?

Shell shock

Artillery attacks could last for days, even weeks, with the trenches being continually shelled causing soldiers to shelter as best they could in dug-outs and deeper shelters. Many soldiers suffered from 'shell shock', whose symptoms included anxiety, nervous tics and severe nightmares. By 1918 there had been over 80,000 cases diagnosed, accounting for nearly 1.3 per cent of all casualties. Initial treatment was to keep the men at the front, give them rest, food and talks to calm them down. If the condition showed no signs of improvement they were sent to hospital. Some hospitals developed specialist centres for treating shell shock.

Illness and disease

Quite apart from wounds, soldiers also experienced outbreaks of illness and disease at the front.

Infection

Infection of the wound was a major reason for death from injury. Bullet and shell fragments carried other material such as pieces of muddy clothing and soil deep into the body which often led to infection. Many soldiers were able to recover from their initial injury but died when infection developed. The infection that caused most deaths was gas **gangrene**, which was carried by bacteria living in soil and was very fast developing. Wounds infected with this bacteria swelled up with gas, turned white, then green and made a bubbling sound when pressed. In the days before antibiotics there was little doctors could do to fight this infection.

Trench fever

Trench fever (pyrexia) was spread by lice which lived in the seams of clothing and in blankets. As lice were common among soldiers at the front, trench fever was widespread. Its symptoms included headaches, shivering and pains in the bones and joints which could last for days. It debilitated soldiers, making them unfit to fight and they sometimes required spells in hospital. Between July 1917 and July 1918, 15 per cent of British soldiers were unfit for duty due to trench fever. To help combat it clothing was disinfected and when soldiers returned from the front line their uniforms were fumigated, washed and ironed.

Trench foot

Trench floors quickly filled with water and mud in rainy conditions and to help stop having to stand in water-logged ground **duckboards** were used. However, these could not prevent a soldier from developing the condition known as trench foot. This was the result of a fungal infection brought on by constant immersion of feet in water, leaving them numb, swollen and blistered, causing them to turn blue from the restriction of blood flow through the foot. The condition deteriorated rapidly and could lead to gangrene. This could then spread to other parts of the body and so the only treatment was usually amputation.

As instances of trench foot became more and more common, medical officers ordered men to change their socks regularly and to rub water repellent whale oil into their feet. The latter did have a major impact as did regular foot inspections of men at the front.

Frostbite

Like trench foot, frostbite, which was caused by exposure to extreme cold, damaged the skin and sometimes muscle tissue. It cut off circulation, usually to the hands and feet, causing fingers, toes and sometimes feet to have to be amputated. In 1917, 21,000 British soldiers were admitted to hospital with frostbite.

Body lice

Body lice, which lived in the uniforms of soldiers and on the skin, was a particular problem. The insects lived off the blood of their hosts and their bites caused intense itching, which could lead to blisters and boils. Sometimes the wounds caused by bites became infected and this could lead to trench fever.

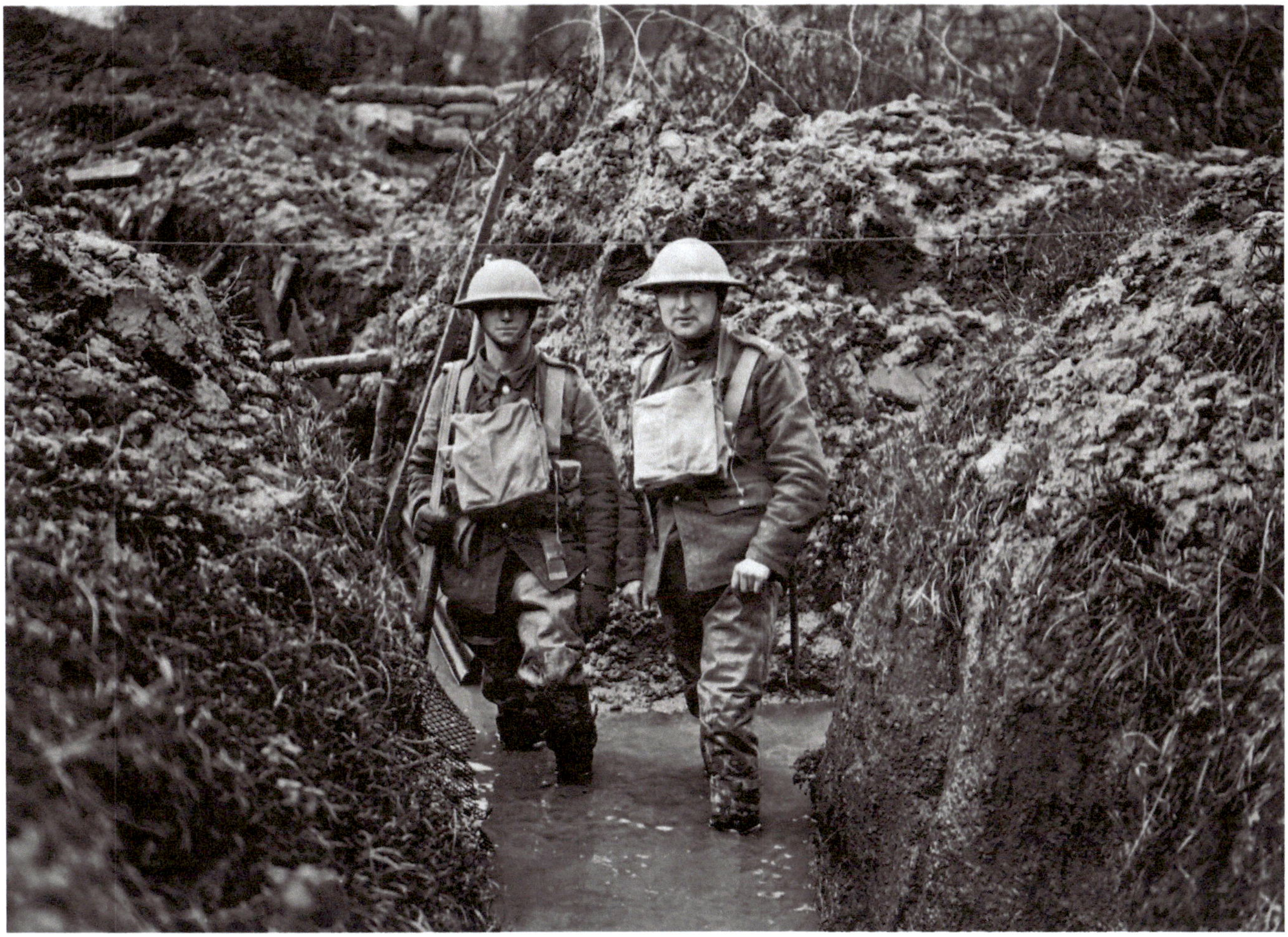

8 Study of a historic environment: the British sector of the Western Front, 1914–18

▲ Source C: British soldiers wading through mud in a trench on the Western Front

> **THINK**
>
> What is the connection in medical terms between Source C and Source D?

> **ACTIVITY**
>
> 'Many of the casualties admitted to field hospitals were suffering not from wounds but from illnesses caught due to the harsh conditions experienced in the trenches.'
>
> Write a report to the chief medical officer of the British Army in support of this statement, supporting your account with references to particular illnesses and diseases.

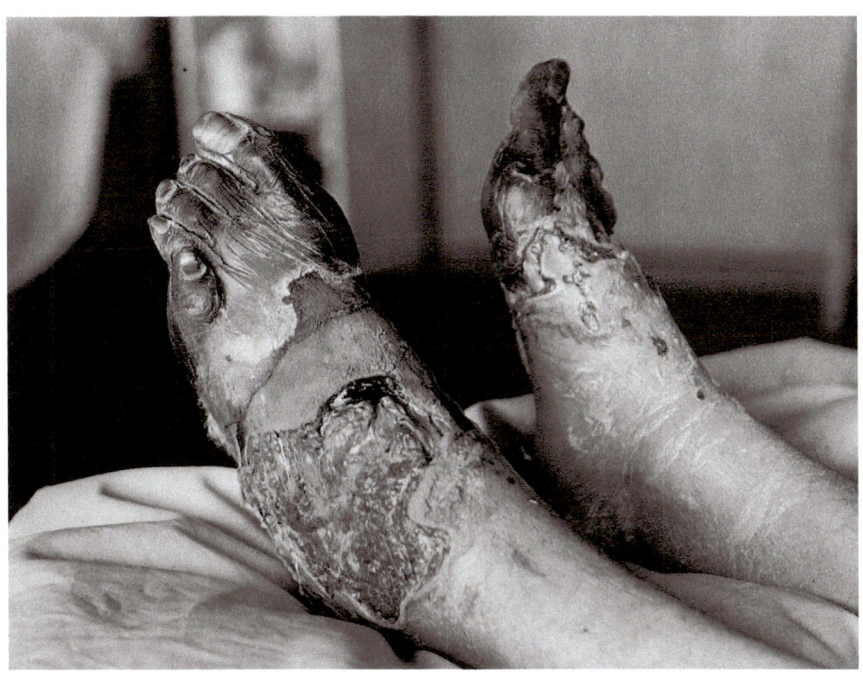

▲ Source D: An extreme incidence of trench foot

Treatment and care of the wounded

On a quiet day a few hundred British soldiers were wounded on the Western Front but during a major offensive or enemy attack the numbers could run into the thousands. A soldier wounded in no-man's land would normally have to wait until it became dark for men from his trench to retrieve him as doing so during the day meant exposing the rescuers to enemy fire. No-man's land and the trenches were difficult areas to move around in, often being deep in mud and littered with shell craters filled with water. Transporting the wounded was therefore extremely hazardous.

> **Source E:** An account of wounded soldiers awaiting medical attention, taken from the diary of Sapper J. Davey of the Royal Engineers written on 10 May 1915
>
> *Not many hours went by before we were shelled out of this position and had to come farther back. I don't know how we have fared in the firing line. We went out at night to put some wire entanglements in front of the trenches. The sights were too awful for words. In our advanced trench when the flares went up we could see how things really were. Numbers of poor fellows lay in the bottom of the trench, the wounded amongst the dead crying for water and the stretcher bearers. Some had been waiting a day and a half to be brought in.*

Processing and treating casualties

The survival of badly wounded soldiers often depended upon prompt medical treatment, something that was not always possible during the midst of battle. Once they had been retrieved and taken to the nearest aid post then, initial treatment was given before they were sent on to the dressing station. The next stage was assessment of the severity of the wound in the casualty clearing station before being sent on to a base hospital or returned to the front, bandaged up.

Regimental aid post and stretcher bearers

The stretcher bearers had the task of recovering men from the battlefield and carrying them, often under fire, to the nearest regimental aid post. Here they received emergency treatment by the stretcher bearers who carried basic medical supplies such as bandages and morphine. There were usually 16 stretcher bearers attached to each battalion of up to 1000 soldiers.

The regimental aid post was often little more than a dug-out in the side of a trench and here the regimental medical officer would determine whether the wounded soldier had been lightly wounded or was in need of more medical treatment. In the case of the latter, he would be sent on to the dressing station.

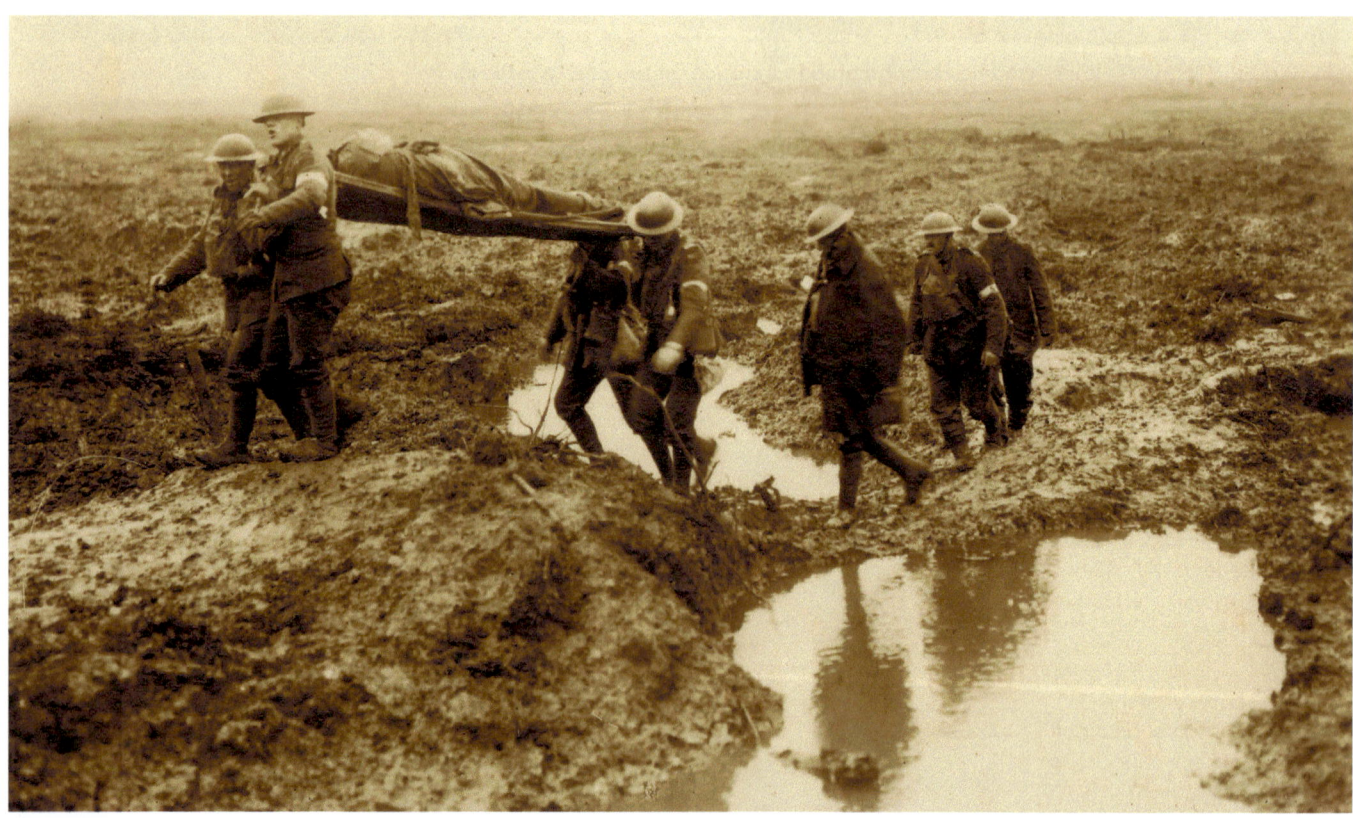

▲ **Source F:** Stretcher bearers of the Royal Army Medical Corp attempting to carry a wounded soldier through the muddy battleground at Passchendaele on 1 August 1917

Field ambulance, dressing station and triage

Field ambulances were mobile medical units often set up in tents or derelict buildings, situated at least a quarter of a mile behind the front line. They served as dressing stations and operated a system of triage, which involved making an initial assessment of the wounded, then sorting them into groups depending upon the severity of the wound. The stations were staffed by medical officers and support staff such as orderlies and nurses. Doctors at dressing stations could do little more than put on bandages or splints and give morphine. Serious cases were passed on to casualty clearing stations by motorised or horse-drawn ambulances.

Casualty clearing station

Casualty clearing stations were situated several miles behind the front line and were based in either wooden huts or tents. They contained a staff of around seven doctors with nurses and other staff such as orderlies, and here doctors carried out surgery in operating theatres. They had access to mobile X-ray machines (see page 118) and wards to accommodate around 50 men. Upon arrival a triage system was operated, dividing the wounded into three groups:

1. less severely wounded to be put on trains and sent to a base hospital
2. those in need of a life-saving operation such as an amputation of a badly damaged limb or the cleaning and sewing up of wounds
3. those beyond medical help who were sent to the 'moribund ward' to be made comfortable in their final hours.

Base hospitals and Blighty

The destination of the seriously wounded was the base hospital, which could be a civilian hospital or a converted building. They were generally situated near railways so patients could be moved quickly. They contained operating theatres, X-ray machines and laboratories for the identification of infections. Some of these hospitals were larger and could accommodate several thousand patients. From here those patients who had a wound that was not severe but bad enough to get them sent back home to Blighty (England) for further treatment and recovery were put on hospital trains heading for the port, or were sent to a recovery ward before being sent back to the front.

The RAMC and the nursing corps

All medical personnel in 1914 belonged to the RAMC – Royal Army Medical Corps. It consisted of all ranks ranging from doctors to ambulance drivers and stretcher bearers. As the war on the Western Front expanded so the RAMC expanded, growing from a staff of 9000 men in 1914 to 113,000 in 1918.

At the start of the war the only nurses allowed to treat soldiers were the well-trained Queen Alexandra's nurses, who numbered just 300 in 1914. However, they had grown to a size of 10,000 by 1918 and had been joined by 15,000 unpaid volunteer nurses. They belonged to the VAD (Voluntary Aid Detachment) and were mainly middle- and upper-class women who had never previously had a job but who now felt the need to nurse the wounded at the front.

By the end of the war over 25,000 women were serving as nurses at the front.

Dates	Lying	Sitting
2 August	88	50
3 August	69	300
4 August	35	452
5 August	31	66
6 August	94	178
7 August	48	109
8 August	28	125
9 August	34	157
10 August	53	86
11 August	113	841
12 August	88	102
13 August	36	112
14 August	22	60
Totals	739	2656
Grand total		3395

▲ Table 8.3: The number of patients who attended the 76th Field Ambulance Advanced Dressing Station at Hooge Chateau between 2 and 14 August 1917

> ### THINK
> 1. Use Source E and your own knowledge to explain the difficulty of attending to the wounded lying in no-man's land.
> 2. What does Table 8.3 tell us about the task facing medical staff working in field ambulance stations?
> 3. How significant was the introduction of a system of triage in improving the treatment of the wounded on the Western Front?

Development of surgical methods and medical innovation

The war helped to push forward advances in medical knowledge and practices. Surgeons pioneered new techniques to treat wounds and injuries. Technological advances, such as the use of blood transfusions and the use of X-rays helped save lives, as did the development of more efficient evacuation of the wounded from the battlefield.

Treating wounds and injuries

The war saw the development of new types of weapons that caused death and injury on a scale not seen in any previous wars. This demanded changes in the way medical staff dealt with and treated soldiers wounded and injured during battle.

Vaccination

Many soldiers in the trenches died from typhus or tetanus. During the first year of the war tetanus infection was the cause of 32 out of every 1000 deaths on the Western Front. From 1915 onwards troops were vaccinated against typhus and tetanus and this reduced the death rate from tetanus to just 2 in every 1000 deaths. As a result vaccination became routine in the post-war years.

Amputations and artificial limbs

Many wounded soldiers had to have limbs amputated to stop the spread of gangrene. While infection was still a problem for the amputee, the war years saw considerable advances in the development of artificial limbs and moving joints. This aided the mobility of the amputee.

Plastic surgery

This was a completely new area of medicine but one which made great advances during the war years. Some soldiers experienced terrible wounds caused by bullet and shell damage, especially to the face. By the end of 1915 seven hospitals in France had specialist areas for dealing with wounds requiring plastic surgery. One man who pioneered the use of plastic surgery was Harold Gillies, a British army surgeon, who developed a specialist department at the Queen's Hospital in Kent to treat facial injuries. It was opened in 1917 and provided over 1000 beds and treated over 2000 soldiers injured in the Battle of the Somme. New techniques were developed by surgeons to rebuild noses with bits of bone taken from a rib, and it was discovered how to graft skin from one part of the body to another.

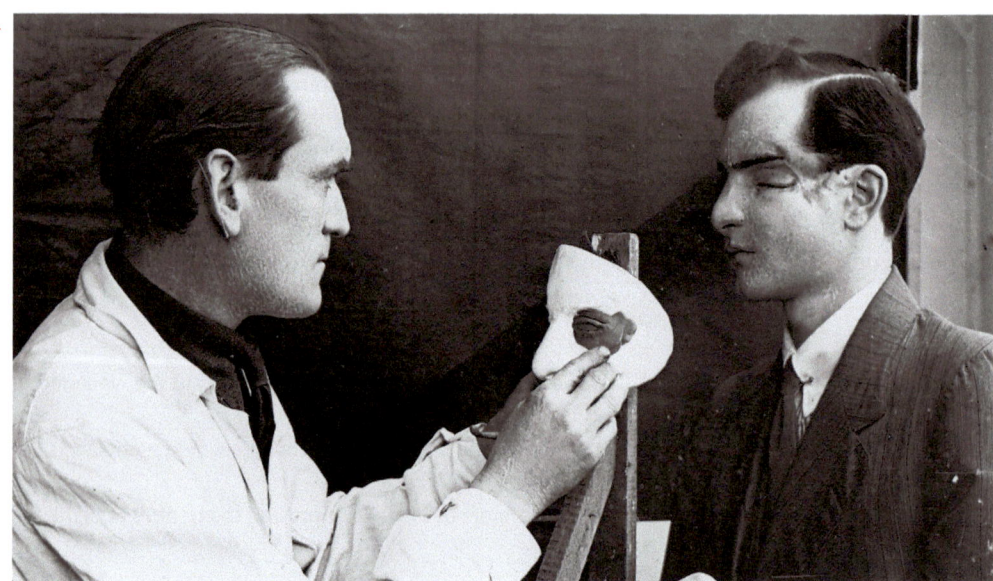

Source G: Captain Wood, an artist before he joined the Army, painting an artificial face plate fixed over the cavity made in the soldier's face by a bullet wound near or in the eye

Brain surgery

The huge number of head and brain injuries pushed surgeons to develop surgical techniques, particularly brain surgery. Two developments helped this process – the ability to undertake blood transfusions and the use of X-rays to locate metal fragments located inside the head. The American surgeon Harvey Cushing invented a surgical magnet to extract bullets from head wounds.

Many surgeons who furthered their skills in battlefield hospitals set up as specialists back home after the war.

The Thomas splint

During the first years of the war over 80 per cent of soldiers who had their femur (thigh bone) broken by gunfire died from their injury. Medical officers had only simple splints which did not stop the broken bone ends from moving, causing blood loss and the onset of infection. An invention in 1916 by the Welsh surgeon, Hugh Owen Thomas, had a dramatic impact, causing the death rate from such an injury to reduce from 80 to 20 per cent.

This invention was the 'Thomas splint'. It was designed to stabilise the fracture, putting the leg lengthways to stop the bones grinding against each other. This greatly reduced blood loss, helped to reduce the risk of infection and resulted in a reduction in the number of amputations required. Thomas' nephew, Robert Jones, who was the British Army's Director of Military Orthopaedics in 1916, made sure the 'Thomas splint' was available for use at the front. The basic design of the 'Thomas' is still in use today.

> **Source H:** An account of brain surgery printed in the *British Medical Journal* in June 1917, written by Surgeon-General Sir Anthony Bowlby
>
> *A primary cleansing of the wound. The transmission of the patient as soon as possible to the hospital where he will convalesce. The taking of X-ray pictures. The excision of the scalp and bone wound. A limited and careful removal of foreign bodies. The covering of the exposed brain. The closure of the wound, with superficial drainage, and prolonged rest in bed.*

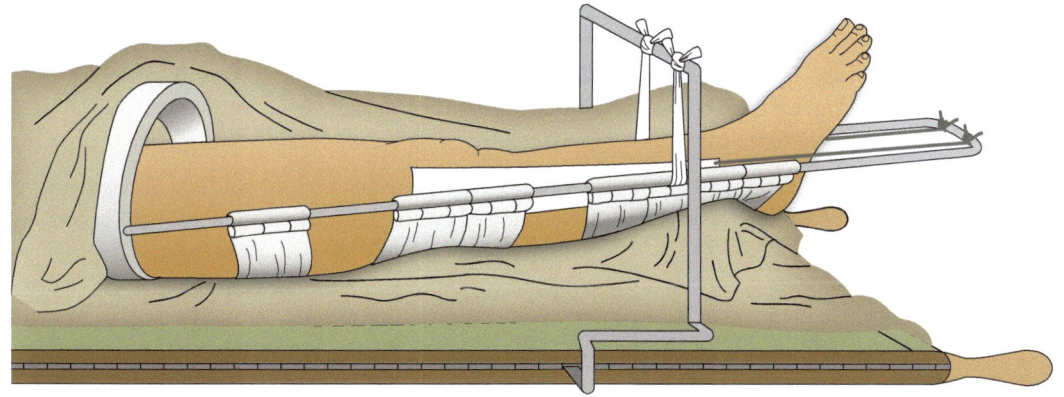

▲ Figure 8.4: The Thomas splint in use

Fighting infection – development of aseptic surgery

One of the biggest causes of death among wounded soldiers was infection. During the late nineteenth century the surgeon Joseph Lister pioneered aseptic surgery, performing surgery under sterile conditions which considerably reduced the onset of infection post-operation (see page 47). By 1914 aseptic surgery was standard procedure in all British hospitals.

However, on the battlefield where surgeons had to operate under less than hygienic conditions, it was difficult to prevent the infection of a wound. The presence of bacteria lodged in dirty clothing was an added problem as this often led to the development of gas gangrene.

It was through trial and error that surgeons attempted of overcome these difficulties. They used chemicals such as carbolic acid and hydrogen peroxide to kill bacteria already in wounds. They discovered that by cutting away infected tissue and soaking the wound with saline solution, infection rates did reduce. They also learnt not to sew up wounds immediately but to keep them open for the use of antiseptics. However, this was only a limited improvement and it was not until the discovery of penicillin just before the Second World War that the problem of infection was really addressed.

> **THINK**
> 1. Study Sources G and H. What do they tell us about advances in surgery during the war years?
> 2. Did the invention of the Thomas splint have much impact upon the successful treatment of leg injuries?

Blood transfusion

Blood transfusions had been tried ever since William Harvey had discovered the circulation of the blood (see page 58) but most patients died shortly afterwards. A major advance was made in 1900 when Karl Landsteiner discovered that blood could be grouped into four types and that each patient needs blood from someone of the same blood group, and that only some blood groups could be mixed together safely. This knowledge meant that the lives of thousands of soldiers were saved on the Western Front through immediate blood transfusions, especially at casualty clearing stations via arm-to-arm transfusions.

> **Source I:** A rifleman, Charlie Shephard, describes giving blood in an arm-to-arm transfusion during the 1914–18 war. His interview was recorded in a book by L. MacDonald, *Roses of No Man's Land* (1980)
>
> I've still got the scar where they opened me up to get the tube into the vein … there it was running into the other chap's left arm. He lost a leg – been down in No Man's Land. Gangrene had set in and they'd had to amputate. Oh, he was like death. As white as a sheet … I was lying watching the other bloke and, believe me, you could see the colour coming back into the man's face.

However, the problem remained that it was not possible to store blood because it clotted so quickly. The demand for blood during wartime made a solution to this problem very urgent. A series of discoveries helped to find a solution. In 1914 an American scientist, Richard Lewisohn, discovered that sodium citrate could be added to blood to stop it clotting and during the war an American army doctor, O. H. Robertson, used this method to keep blood fresh so it could be used to help British soldiers. Scientists also discovered that keeping blood refrigerated allowed it to be stored for longer periods and in 1917 a British surgeon, Geoffrey Keynes, developed a portable machine that could store blood to enable transfusions to be carried out more easily.

These advances in blood transfusions saved the lives of thousands of soldiers at the front. By the time of the Second World War all developed countries had set up their own blood banks.

Portable X-rays

The scientist William Rontgen first discovered X-rays in 1895 but it was during the First World War that they really became important. It was soon realised that X-rays could help to save lives by allowing for the speedy location of bullets, shrapnel and tiny fragments of metal in the body of a wounded soldier, enabling surgeons to locate them easily and thereby reducing the chances of infection which was a common cause of death. The problem however, was that there were very few X-ray machines before 1914 and fewer still were portable enough to be used on the battlefield.

One of the pioneers in radiography was Marie Curie and at the start of the war she temporarily gave up her work at the Radium Institute in Paris to concentrate upon developing a portable X-ray machine. By October 1914 she had constructed the first of 20 radiology vehicles which transported portable X-ray machines to the front line. By 1916 most casualty clearing stations and hospitals had X-ray equipment and they became standard equipment in post-war hospitals.

> **THINK**
>
> 'The ability to carry out blood transfusions and the use of x-ray machines helped save the lives of thousands of soldiers wounded on the Western Front.' What evidence could you put forward to justify this statement?

The significance of advances in the treatment and care of the wounded

The First World War proved to be a catalyst for medical improvement. It speeded up developments in medicine resulting from discoveries made in the nineteenth century, such as the discovery of blood types which facilitated the development of blood transfusion. The war also forced developments in surgery, particularly in the field of plastic surgery, and in the development of new technology such as portable X-ray machines. What was significant was the pace of change – a soldier wounded in 1918 had a much greater chance of survival than one who had been wounded in 1914.

> **ACTIVITIES**
>
> Working in pairs, study the diagram below.
>
> 1. In your opinion, which of the five developments identified in the diagram was the most significant in achieving improvements in medical care?
> 2. Justify your choice to the rest of the class.

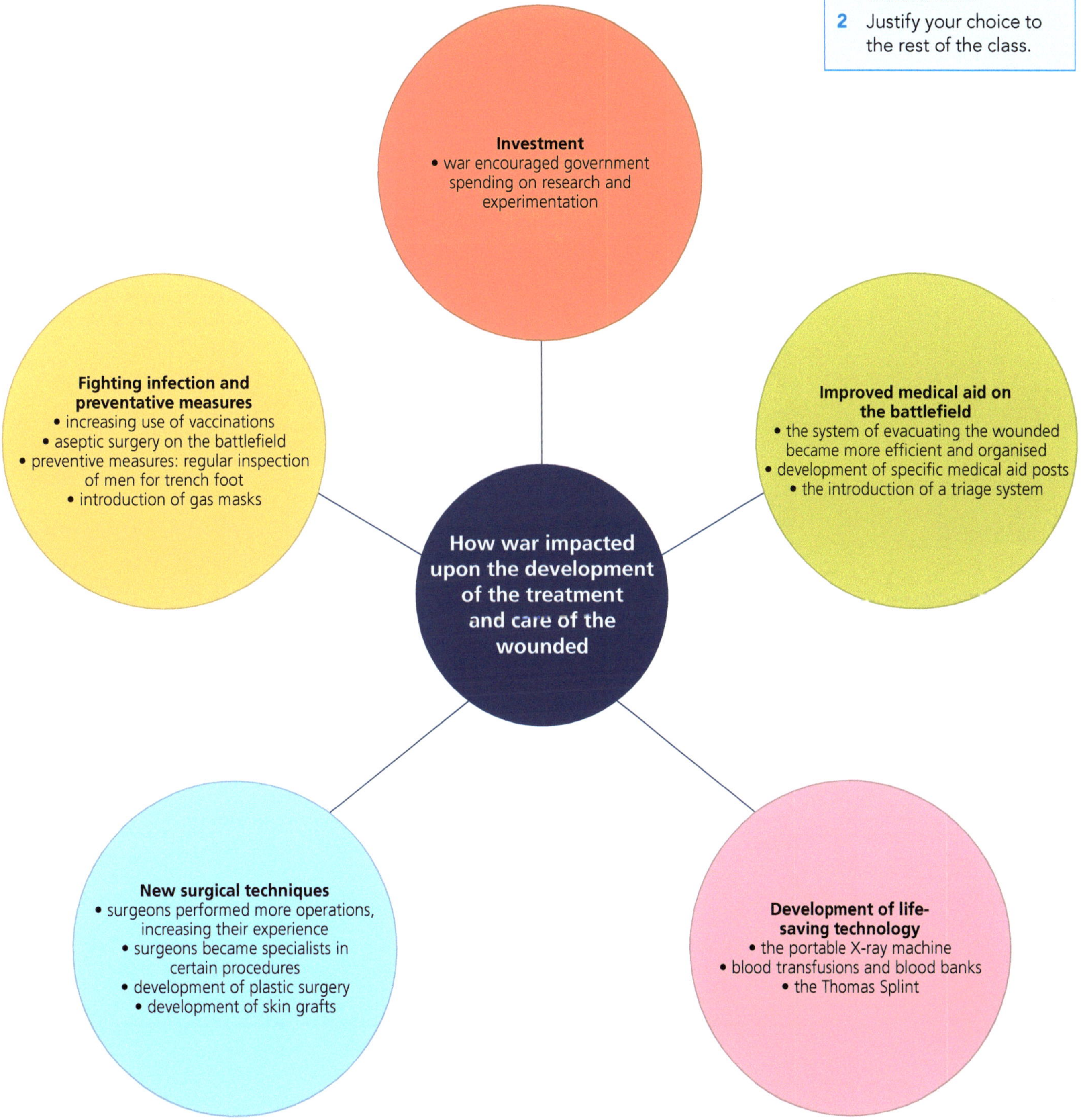

How war impacted upon the development of the treatment and care of the wounded

Investment
- war encouraged government spending on research and experimentation

Fighting infection and preventative measures
- increasing use of vaccinations
- aseptic surgery on the battlefield
- preventive measures: regular inspection of men for trench foot
- introduction of gas masks

Improved medical aid on the battlefield
- the system of evacuating the wounded became more efficient and organised
- development of specific medical aid posts
- the introduction of a triage system

New surgical techniques
- surgeons performed more operations, increasing their experience
- surgeons became specialists in certain procedures
- development of plastic surgery
- development of skin grafts

Development of life-saving technology
- the portable X-ray machine
- blood transfusions and blood banks
- the Thomas Splint

▲ Figure 8.5: Impact of the First World War on the development of treatment and care for the wounded

FOCUS TASK REVISITED

Look back over the focus task you have completed while working through this chapter.
1. What, in your opinion, was the biggest problem facing medical staff working in the trenches?
2. How successfully was the problem overcome?
3. Which of the medical advances you have studied in this chapter has had the biggest long-term impact upon the methods and procedures used to treat and care for the wounded in battle?

TOPIC SUMMARY

- The First World War was fought between 1914 and 1918.
- The war on the Western Front was very different to previous wars – it was a static, attritional war.
- Both sides were unable to defeat the other in battle and the result was stalemate.
- Both sides dug in, constructing lines of trenches, the land between enemy trenches being termed 'no-man's land'.
- Large battles, such as the Marne, Ypres, the Somme and Cambrai, resulted in a high death rate and an equally high casualty rate.
- High casualty rates were the result of trench warfare and the new more powerful weapons developed to fight this new type of warfare – artillery shells, gas shells and machine guns.
- Conditions for soldiers spending time in the trenches were difficult and resulted in illnesses and disease such as trench fever, trench foot, body lice, frostbite.
- New systems were developed to cope with having to treat the high numbers of men wounded at the front.
- A series of medical aid posts were established and a system of triage was put in place to determine which medical post a wounded soldier needed to be sent to.
- New surgical methods were pioneered to treat the terrible wounds and this led to the development of new specialisms such as brain surgery and plastic surgery.
- The invention of new machines and equipment such as the Thomas splint and the use of portable X-rays had a major impact upon improving the chances of survival for wounded soldiers.
- There were developments in the methods to reduce the risk of infection – vaccination, aseptic surgery and blood transfusions, all of which had a long-term impact upon the treatment of the wounded in battle.
- The war pushed forward the pace of medical improvement.

Practice questions

1. Describe two main features of medical advances in tending the wounded on the Western Front.
2. Explain how the environment of the Western Front during the First World War was significant in bringing about change in the methods used to combat illness and disease during the twentieth century.

Guidance for the Eduqas Examination

Examination guidance for Question 1

This section provides guidance on how to answer the 'similarity and difference' question. You will have to pick out information from three sources to identify both similarities and differences. Look at the following question:

> Look at the three sources below which show the treatment of illness over time. Use Sources A, B and C to identify one similarity and one difference in the treatment of illness over time.

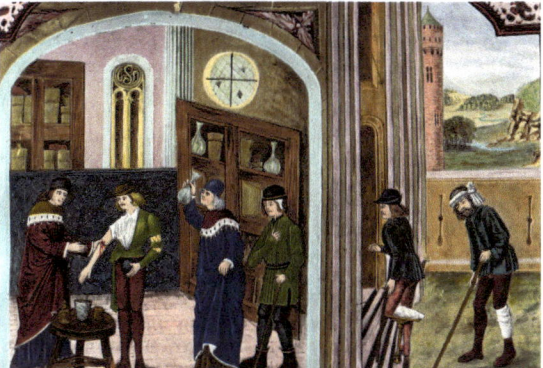

▲ **Source A:** A man being bled using leeches during medieval times

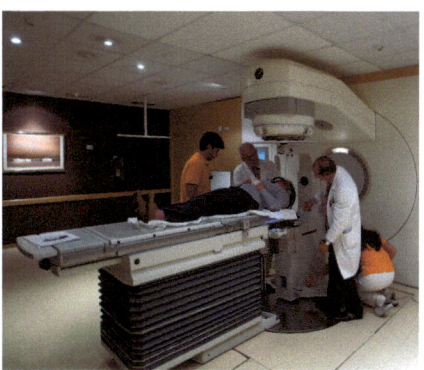

▲ **Source C:** A patient undergoing radiation therapy

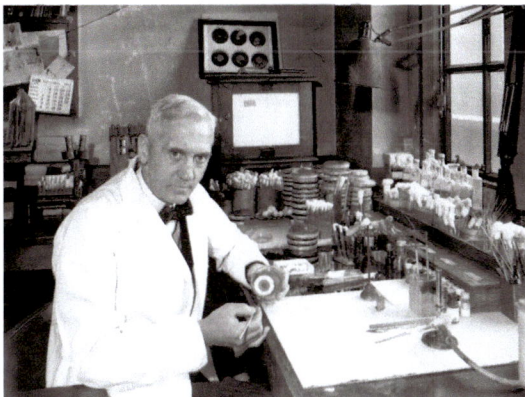

▲ **Source B:** Professor Alexander Fleming and Penicillin

How to answer

- Study the three sources – pick out features that are the same or similar.
- Pick out points that contrast – which show things that are different.
- Make sure you refer to both similarity **and** difference in your answer.

WJEC Eduqas GCSE History: Changes in health and medicine in Britain, c.500 to the present day

Example

Step 1: Identify features of similarity – things which are the same across the sources

All the sources show attempts by medical persons to treat illness. Within their own time period they were all considered to be medical experts – Source A shows a barber surgeon, Source B a professor of medicine and Source C a specialist doctor.

Step 2: Identify features of difference – things which contrast and are not the same across the sources

However, the sources differ in the type of treatment shown. Source A shows primitive methods of bleeding the patient. Source B shows the development of specialist drugs to fight illness and disease, and Source C shows the use of modern scanning machines to detect illness and disease.

Now try answering the following question:

Look at the three sources below, which show public health over time. Use Sources A, B and C to identify one similarity and one difference in public health over time.

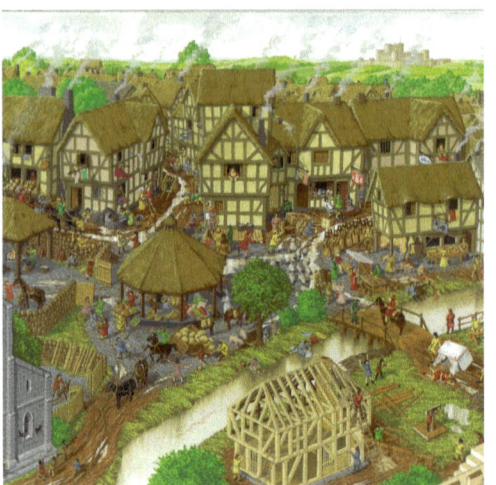

▲ **Source A:** A medieval town scene

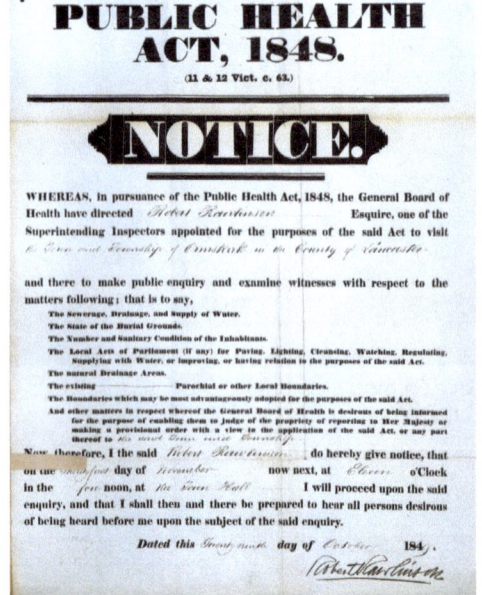

▲ **Source B:** The Public Health Act 1848

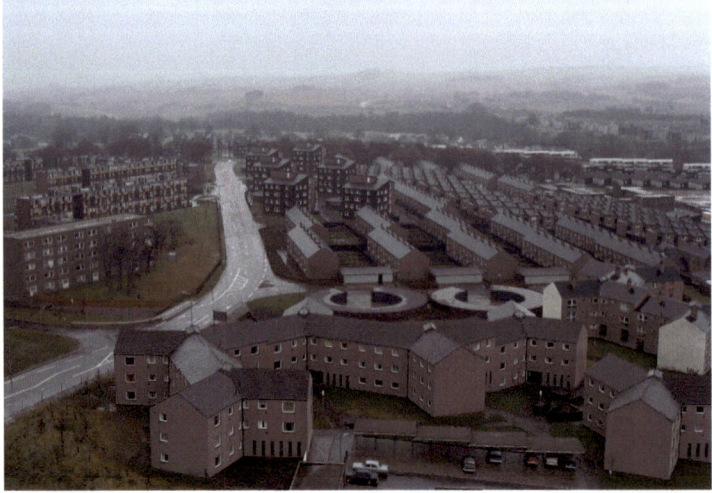

▲ **Source C:** A housing development of the 1970s

Guidance for the Eduqas Examination

Examination guidance for Question 2

This section provides guidance on how to answer the 'reliability' question. You will need to analyse and evaluate the reliability of two sources. Look at the following question:

> Which of the two sources is the more reliable to a historian studying the development of vaccination during the late eighteenth and early nineteenth centuries?

Source D: Extract from Dr Edward Jenner's book *An Enquiry into the causes and effects of Variola Vaccinae, known by the name of Cowpox*, which was published in 1798

Case 17 James Phipps

I selected a healthy boy, about eight years old. The matter was taken from the [cowpox] sore on the hand of Sarah Nelmes and it was inserted on 14 May 1796 into the boy by two cuts each about half an inch long. On the seventh day he complained of uneasiness, on the ninth he became a little chilly, lost his appetite and had a slight headache and spent the night with some degree of restlessness, but on the following day he was perfectly well.

In order to ascertain that the boy was secure from the contagion of the smallpox, he was inoculated with smallpox matter, but no disease followed.

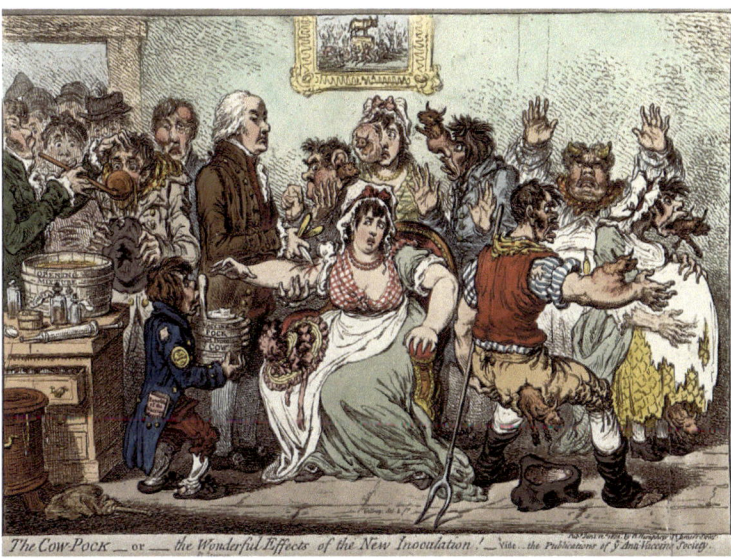

▲ **Source E:** A cartoon drawn by James Gillray which was given the title *The Cowpox – or – the Wonderful Effects of the New Inoculation*. It was published in 1802 and shows people's panic over the new process of vaccination

How to answer

- You need to make sure you refer to both the content and the author of each source.
- Study the content of Source D and use your knowledge to make a judgement about:
  - ☐ the accuracy of what is said or shown in the source
  - ☐ whether the tone of the writing or the style of the picture give a clue as to its reliability.
- Study the author of Source D. What information does the attribution give you to make a judgement about reliability? Look at:
  - ☐ who wrote/produced it
  - ☐ when it was written/produced
  - ☐ whether the title provides a clue as to its reliability
  - ☐ who the source was aimed at; does the intended audience have an impact upon reliability.
- Repeat the same process for Source E.
- Conclude with a judgement – which of the two sources is the most reliable and why.

WJEC Eduqas GCSE History: Changes in health and medicine in Britain, *c.*500 to the present day

Example

Step 1: Explain the content of Source D and link it to your knowledge of the topic area. Make and support judgements about the reliability of the author.

> Source D is reliable to a historian because it is an extract from the case notes of Edward Jenner which was included in his book *An Enquiry into the causes and effects of Variola Vaccinae, known by the name of Cowpox*. This book was published in 1798 and it contains Jenner's research findings into his experiments with inoculation with cowpox and smallpox. In his account he describes how in 1796 he injected a small boy, James Phipps, with the pus from the sores of a milkmaid with cowpox. Phipps developed cowpox and he recovered. He was then given a dose of smallpox, but he did not develop smallpox. Jenner provides a fact-based account of his work which makes it reliable to the historian as it outlines, without any apparent bias, how he carried out his experiments with inoculation. This makes it very useful to the historian.

Step 2: Explain the content of Source E and link it to your knowledge of the topic area. Make and support judgements about the reliability of the author.

> Source E is considerably less reliable as it is a humorous cartoon produced by the famous cartoonist James Gillray in 1802. It is a contemporary reflection upon attitudes towards Jenner's work. It shows people in a panic about the idea of injecting a person with cowpox and the effects it could have upon them. The cartoonist has highlighted the level of concern that existed to the idea of inoculation and vaccination by drawing parts of cows growing out of the arms and heads of some of the people who have already been vaccinated. While the cartoon was intended to entertain and therefore exaggerates the level of concern, it does reflect the reality of the opposition which faced Jenner. People did object to inoculation due to a belief that people would turn into cows. The source is reliable to the historian in part as it provides evidence of opposition to inoculation and vaccination but it does not reflect in any accurate way the actual effects of inoculation.

Step 3: Conclude with a final reasoned judgement – which of the two sources is the most reliable and why.

> Of the two sources, Source D is clearly the more reliable to the historian studying the development of vaccination as it is based on fact. It records the research notes of one of the pioneers of vaccination. Source E has little reliability as it is humorous and what it actually shows is not reality. However it can still be useful in mirroring contemporary concerns and the arguments that were put forward against vaccination.

Now try to answer the following question:

Which of the two sources is more reliable to a historian studying the methods of treating illness and disease during the eighteenth and nineteenth centuries?

Source D: Extract from a book by Joseph Lister, *On the New Method of Treating Compound Fracture*, which was published in 1867

A piece of lint dipped in carbolic acid was laid on the wound, and splints padded with cotton wool were applied. It was left undisturbed for four days and, when examined, it showed no signs of suppuration [discharge/pus]. For the next four days the wound was dressed with lint soaked with a solution of water and carbolic acid and olive oil which further prevented irritation to the skin. No pus was present and at the end of six weeks I found the bones united and I discarded the splints. The sore was entirely healed.

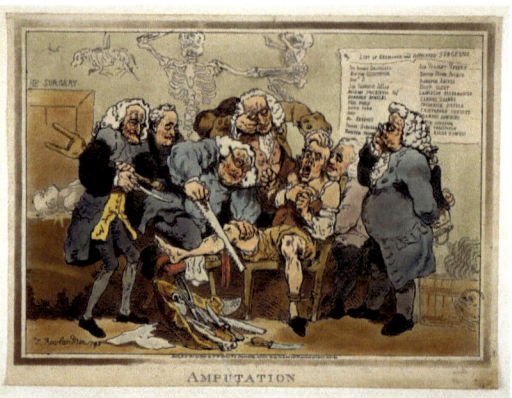

▲ **Source E:** A cartoon drawn by Thomas Rowlandson in 1793 showing an operation before the use of anaesthetics was available

Examination guidance for Question 3

This section provides guidance on how to answer a 'describe' question. You will have to demonstrate your own knowledge and understanding of a key feature. Look at the following question:

> Describe the development of methods used to combat the spread of the plague during the Black Death.

How to answer

- You need to identify and describe at least two key features.
- Only include information that is directly relevant.
- Be specific; avoid generalised comments.

Example

Step 1: Identify and develop a key reason/feature, supporting it with specific detail.

> The Black Death spread rapidly across Europe during 1348–49 causing the death of up to 40 per cent of the population. It was highly contagious and various methods were developed to try and prevent its spread. One common method was that of quarantine. Travellers were placed in quarantine zones before being allowed to enter a town. Another method adopted to stop the spread of disease from dead bodies awaiting individual burial was to speed up the process by taking the dead away to be buried in one large plague pit outside the town walls. They needed to be buried as quickly as possible. Infected families had to board up doors and windows to prevent infecting neighbours.

Step 2: Identify and develop other key reasons/features. Aim to cover two to three reasons/features in some detail.

> Other methods developed included the increasing use of potions like theriac or the carrying of scented flowers and herbs, in the belief that they would kill off the plague. The clothes of diseased people were burnt in the hope it would kill off the infection. In an attempt to appeal to God for salvation flagellants whipped themselves in a display of suffering, hoping this penance would cause the disease to pass them by. In an attempt to stop catching the plague doctors developed protective clothing, wearing gowns and hoods when making house calls, their hood containing a beak which was stuffed with herbs.

> **Now try to answer the following question:**
> Describe the development of the theory of the four humours during the medieval period.

Examination guidance for Question 4

This section provides tips on how to answer the 'explain why' question. You have to identify a number of reasons to explain why a key development/issue was important or significant. Look at the following question:

> Explain why the work of Pasteur and Koch was important in the advancement of medical knowledge during the nineteenth and twentieth centuries.

How to answer

- You should aim to give a variety of explained reasons.
- Try to include specific details such as names, dates, events, developments and consequences.
- Always support your statements with examples.
- Remember that you need to provide a judgement, evaluating the importance or significance of the named individual, development or issue.

Example

Step 1: Provide several reasons to support the view that the factor mentioned in the question was important/significant. Include specific factual detail to support your judgement.

> The work of Louis Pasteur and Robert Koch was very important in the development of medical knowledge in the nineteenth and twentieth centuries. Pasteur developed the 'germ theory,' which suggested that germs were the cause of disease. Through examining the causes of diseases he discovered that the process of heating liquids helped to kill germs, a process that came to be known as pasteurisation. Pasteur went on to develop vaccines for diseases like chicken cholera, anthrax and rabies, and experimented in methods of vaccination and immunisation. His research had a significant impact upon the treatment of illness.

Step 2: Make sure you provide a reasoned judgement upon the degree of importance/significance. Make links to the longer-term impact.

> Koch developed Pasteur's work further by isolating the bacteria responsible for TB, cholera and anthrax. He pioneered the new science of bacteriology, proving that a specific germ caused a specific disease, and in 1905 he was awarded the Nobel Prize for his research work. Through their experiments with germs, both Pasteur and Koch played a very important and significant role in the development of medical knowledge. Later scientists were able to use their methods to develop a vaccine for diphtheria and syphilis.

> **Now try to answer the following question:**
> Explain why the work of Edwin Chadwick was important in the improvement of public health in the nineteenth and twentieth centuries.

Examination guidance for Question 5

This section provides guidance on how to answer the 'outline question'. You need to explain how and why the key issue named in the question has changed/developed over time. Look at the following question:

> Outline how the methods of caring for patients have improved between c.500 and the present day.

How to answer

- Make sure your answer covers three historical time periods – the medieval, early modern and modern eras.
- Include specific factual detail such as names, dates, key methods/developments.
- Start a new paragraph for each time period.
- Aim to write roughly equal amounts for each time period.
- Make regular links to the question, evaluating the degree of progress, change or improvement.
- Check your spelling, punctuation and grammar for accuracy.

Example

Step 1: Introduce the topic area to be analysed and discussed in the answer.

> The care and treatment of patients has changed significantly over the centuries. At some times the pace of change has been faster, particularly in recent centuries and, generally speaking, these changes have resulted in an overall improvement in the quality of care provided for patients.

Step 2: Select one time period and discuss the state of medical provision at that time. Provide specific factual detail and make links to the question.

> During the medieval period the body that was mainly responsible for caring for sick people, older people and those in need of medical attention was the church. Over 1100 hospitals were set up across England and Wales during the medieval period, most of them attached to monasteries. Most monasteries had infirmaries which tended to sick people but they were not hospitals like the ones we have today. They provided a place of 'hospitality' which was a place of rest and recuperation rather than a place to be cured from illness or disease. Some specialised in looking after certain types of peoples such as lepers, unmarried pregnant women, young orphaned children and older people. They did not treat sick people but aimed to make patients as comfortable as they could. People who were seriously ill and in need of constant care were often not allowed into the hospital. Life in the hospital was very religion based and patients were expected to spend a proportion of their time praying to God for forgiveness of their sins, the belief being that it was their sinfulness that had caused their illness. During this period the quality of the care was not based upon treating the nature of the illness but upon saving the soul of the patient.

WJEC Eduqas GCSE History: Changes in health and medicine in Britain, *c*.500 to the present day

Step 3: Select a second time period and discuss the improvements/changes in some detail. Make links to the previous time period to show the improvements/changes or lack of improvements/ changes that had taken place.

> A change in the quality and type of care offered to patients began to take place during the early modern period. The decision by Henry VIII to dissolve the monasteries in the 1530s seriously reduced the number of hospitals, which resulted in the church no longer playing the leading role in caring for sick people. During the sixteenth and seventeenth centuries this role was taken on by voluntary charities and individuals. Although these charities were often religion based, endowing hospitals such as St Bartholomew's, St Thomas' and St Mary's in London, their role and function in caring for sick people changed. Even some towns outside London, such as Norwich and Cambridge, set up endowed voluntary hospitals. These institutions were developed further during the eighteenth century by being supported with endowments granted by wealthy individuals such as Thomas Guy and John Addenbrooke, which resulted in the founding of Guy's hospital in London in 1724 and Addenbrooke's hospital in Cambridge in 1766. These institutions marked a turning point in the development of patient care. They employed doctors to treat patients and nurses to care for them on wards. They also issued medicine. This was a significant improvement upon the type of care offered during the medieval period.

Step 4: Select a third time period and discuss the improvements/changes in some detail. Make links to the previous time periods to show the improvements/ changes or lack of improvements/changes that had taken place.

> During the nineteenth century the major developments in patient care were the building of purpose-built hospitals such as Great Ormond Street in 1852, the development of surgical procedures, the advancement of medical knowledge and the creation of a professional nursing staff. Of these the one which had a dramatic impact upon the quality of patient care was the work of Florence Nightingale, who pioneered new methods of nursing. Upon her return from treating the wounded soldiers in the Crimean War Florence set up the Nightingale School of Nursing. This created a professional nursing corps, a move which revolutionised how patients were looked after in hospital. Florence was also heavily involved in the design of new hospitals. As the twentieth century dawned the government began to take on some of the responsibility for tending to sick and injured people. The 1911 National Insurance Scheme devised by Lloyd George enabled members to receive medical treatment if they contributed into the National Insurance Scheme. The Beveridge Report of 1942 forced the government to take on a more direct control of looking after the nation's health and in 1948 the National Health Service was created. This was a radical change which brought about significant improvement in the care of patients, particularly as it now meant patients received free treatment in return for a compulsory National Insurance contribution.

Step 5: Write a conclusion which contains a reasoned judgement upon the question. Remember to check through your answer for correct spelling, punctuation and grammar.

> The biggest change in patient care over the centuries has been a move away from just caring for patients to actually treating the nature of their illness or injury. There has also been a move away from private institutions such as the church or voluntary charities fulfilling the role of providing patient care to the state taking on that role, the result being the creation of the Welfare State and a National Health Service.

Now try to answer the following question:
Outline how attempts to treat illness and disease have improved between c.500 and the present day.

Examination guidance for Question 6(a)

This section provides guidance on how to answer another 'describe' question where you have to demonstrate your knowledge and understanding of a key feature. Look at the following queston:

> Describe two main consequences of the visit of the Great Plague to Eyam in 1665–66.

How to answer

- You need to identify and describe two key features.
- Only include information that is directly relevant.
- Be specific; avoid generalised comments.

Example

Step 1: Identify and develop a key reason/feature, supporting it with specific factual detail.

> A major consequence of the visit of the Great Plague to Eyam was the extreme loss of life. In 1665 Eyam's population stood at around 800 people and by the autumn of 1666 it had been reduced by at least one third. The months of July and August 1666 witnessed the high point of the epidemic with 134 deaths recorded. In total over 260 people in Eyam died as a result of the plague. The loss of life had a dramatic impact upon the lives of those who survived, all of whom had lost family members.

Step 2: Identify and develop a second key reason/feature, supporting it with specific factual detail.

> A second major consequence was the impact this high death toll had on the local economy. Seventy-six families were affected by the plague, some paying a very high price. All the members of the Thorpe family died out, leaving their farm empty and the land uncultivated for some time. The Talbot family was almost wiped out, the only exception being a son who was working away from the village at the time. He later returned to take over the smithy which had stood idle since his father's death. It took the village many years to recover economically from the impact of the plague.

> **Now try to answering the following question:**
> Describe two main causes of the rapid spread of the Great Plague in Eyam, 1665–66.

Examination guidance for Question 6(b)

This section provides guidance on how to answer another 'explain why' question. It is related to the historic environment part of the specification. You have to identify reasons why the historical site you have studied was significant in influencing changes and developments in health and medicine. Look at the following question:

> Explain why the environment of Eyam during the Great Plague was significant in influencing methods used to limit the spread of disease in the seventeenth century.

How to answer

- Identify a number of key reasons which demonstrate change/improvement in health and medicine.
- Discuss each reason in some detail, supporting it with specific factual detail.
- Explain how and why the environment under study brought about such changes.
- Consider the impact of such changes – did they secure improvement/advancement?
- Conclude with a reasoned judgement, making clear links to the question.

Example

Step 1: Introduce the topic under discussion, providing historical context to outline the type of environment being studied.

> An analysis of the environment of Eyam during the Great Plague of 1665–66 reveals that it was partially significant in influencing methods used to limit the spread of disease in the seventeenth century. One of the biggest concerns was the highly contagious nature of the disease which spread at a rapid rate and resulted in a high death rate among infected persons. There was also the impact this had upon the removal and prompt burial of the dead. The methods adopted by the villagers at Eyam in Derbyshire to tackle these problems did show that it was possible to limit the rate of infection and contain disease within a controlled area.

Step 2: Discuss one element of change in some detail, explaining how the environment helped cause the change/improvement.

> The Great Plague of 1665 had it biggest impact in London. The first reported death occurred in April and by July the Plague had spread across the whole city. During September over 26,000 people died. The most pressing problem facing the authorities was how to limit the spread and contain the outbreak. The disease first reached Eyam in August 1665 following the arrival of a parcel of cloth from London which was infected with rat fleas carrying the deadly Black Death disease. By early September the first deaths were recorded in the village. This caused many of the wealthy inhabitants to leave, possibly taking the disease with them, which was a concern to neighbouring settlements.

Guidance for the Eduqas Examination

Step 3: Discuss other features of the environment which caused change in medical procedures, evaluating their significance and importance.

> Medical knowledge about how the disease was spread was limited and there was no known cure. Some people carried sweet-smelling flowers in the belief they would kill off bad-smelling air, while others bought herbal medicines, but they had no real impact. A more successful method was that of imposing isolation, boarding up windows and doors in order to confine infected families within the house. As the plague spread through Eyam during the early spring of 1666, two clerics, William Mompesson and Thomas Stanley, decided to take the lead and they persuaded the villagers to impose a quarantine zone around the village. The immediate impact of this was to stop the spread of the plague to neighbouring villages.

Step 4: Continue to discuss other features of the environment which caused change in medical procedures, evaluating their significance and importance.

> What made the quarantine zone effective was the fact that all the villagers agreed to follow it. It was decided that all persons who died of the plague were to be buried as quickly and as near to their homes as possible in order to reduce the risk of contamination to others. The church was locked and all services were to be held in the open, again to reduce contamination within confined spaces. A quarantine zone was placed around the village. Food supplies from neighbouring villages were left at agreed boundary posts and money was deposited in pans of water or vinegar to try and reduce the risk of infection.
>
> While the death rate in Eyam was high, a consequence of the quarantine was that it stopped the spread of the disease to the nearby settlements of Bakewell, Buxton and Chesterfield. The disease was successfully contained but at a high cost to the villagers of Eyam. Several families were completely wiped out and many experienced the loss of many family members. Of the Hawksworth family, only the wife, Jane, survived out of an extended family of 25.

Step 5: Conclude with a reasoned judgement, demonstrating how the environment under study resulted in changes in health and medicine.

> The important lesson that was gained from the events in Eyam was that the introduction of an enforced quarantine zone could serve as an effective means of stopping the spread of disease. The quick disposal of the dead together with the decision to bury them as close to the actual spot of death also helped to reduce infection rates. The banning of meetings in confined spaces such as the church also helped to limit the risk of infection. When the plague and other highly infectious diseases occurred in later centuries the lessons of what had been done at Eyam to limit the spread of disease were acted upon.

Now try to answer the following question:

Explain why the environment of Eyam during the Great Plague was significant in demonstrating effective ways of containing the spread of disease in the seventeenth century.

Glossary

Allied forces   the armies of countries bound together by formal promises of support

anaesthetics   something used to lessen pain

anticyclone   an area of high atmospheric pressure, in which the air sinks; often winds are light

apothecaries   people who prepare and sell medicines

astrology   study of the planets and the stars to decide what actions to take

barber-surgeons   medieval doctors who performed surgery; they often acted as barbers too!

Boer War   the (Second) Boer War (1899–1902) between Britain and Boers of South Africa over control of the territories (and their gold and diamond deposits) that would later become South Africa

Book of Common Prayer   contained the orders of church services

chiropodist   someone who specialises in looking after feet

cordon sanitaire   an area around a place that prevents a person from entering or leaving

cut-purse   a pickpocket or thief. In the medieval period money was often carried in a purse (a small bag or pouch attached to a belt); the thief would cut the purse free and escape

duckboards   wooden planks laid at the bottom of a trench to form a floor over wet or muddy ground

emetic   a medicine designed to make the patient vomit

four humours   Ancient Greek belief that the body was made up of four body fluids, and that people became ill when these humours were out of balance

gangrene   decay of a part of a person's body because blood has stopped flowing there

Great Exhibition   the first of a series of world fairs exhibiting advances in industry. It was housed in the purpose built Crystal Palace, a huge temporary glass and steel structure

gout   form of arthritis when joints, such as feet, ankles or toes, become inflamed. Often thought to be caused by heavy drinking

heredity   inheriting a disease or illness from parents or grandparents

homeopathy   a system of alternative medicine, based on healing people with natural substances rather than chemical medicines

indulgence   if you bought an indulgence from the church, the church would lessen the punishment for your sins, allowing you to get to heaven more quickly when you died

infant mortality   the number of children who die, usually measured per thousand of the population – for example, infant mortality might be 100 per thousand

inoculation   early form of vaccination where the skin is scratched rather than injected

laissez-faire   a belief that some things were not the job of government, but should be 'left alone' or left to individuals to do for themselves

latrines   toilets

life expectancy   how long, on average, people might expect to live

ligature   a cord used to tie something very tightly, in this case in order to stop bleeding

nationalisation   take over something by government, so government runs the service, factory or industry

nostrums   medical potions which did not prove to be very effective

Oath of Conformity   a vow taken by priests to obey and follow the rules of the church

orderly   an attendant in a hospital who carries out non-medical care

osteopathy   form of treating disease by manipulating bones and muscles

Ottoman Empire   Based on Turkey, with its capital of Constantinople, the Ottoman Empire controlled much of the Mediterranean area from around 1300 until 1922

pandemic   disease covering a huge area or the whole world

poultice   a soft, moist mass of material, often made from bran, flour, herbs, and so on, applied to the body to relieve soreness and inflammation and kept in place with a cloth

Puritan   an extreme Protestant, one who believed in plain, simple church services

Renaissance   meaning rebirth or renewal, usually refers to the period from the fourteenth to seventeenth centuries when great advances were made in learning, science and art.

Royal Society   set up in 1660 by Charles II, this is the national organisation for science and learning. It was designed to promote changes in scientific knowledge

Schlieffen Plan   a military plan of attack devised by German generals to avoid a two-front war against France and Russia; it involved the German army advancing through Belgium to attack France at its weakest point

secular   not to do with religion

septicaemia blood poisoning by infection

sterile free from bacteria or other living micro-organisms; totally clean

triage quick examination of patients to decide priority of treatment

vaccination injection of a mild form of a disease to stop you getting a more dangerous version of the disease

Welfare State introduced after the Second World War, this provided a free health service, unemployment support, council housing and free secondary education

World Health Organization set up by the United Nations in 1948, the WHO aims to improve public health across the whole world

Index

accidental death 16, 24
acupuncture 52
AIDS 27-8
air pollution 90
alchemy 32, 56
almshouses 65, 67
alternative medicine 52
amputations 116
anaesthetics 9, 46
antibodies 40
antiseptics 47-8
apothecaries 44
asthma 45
astrology 43, 56
Attlee, Clement 89

Bacon, Roger 56
bacterial diseases 25-8
bacteriology 40
barber-surgeons 44
Barnard, Christian 51
Bevan, Aneurin 77-8
Beveridge Report 76
Birmingham 88
Black Death 21, 30-1, 95
Black Rats 95
bleeding, as treatment 10, 43
blood, circulation of 58
blood transfusions 118
body lice 112
Booth, Charles 89
brain surgery 117
bubonic plague 94
Burton, Robert 45

Cadwaladr, Betsi 73
cancer treatment 51
casualties, Western Front 114-15
causes of ill health
    accidental death 16
    famine 15
    medieval beliefs 17-21
    poverty 14
    warfare 16
Chadwick, Edwin 84
Chain, Ernest 50
Chamberlain, Joseph 88
Chamberland, Charles 48
Charles II 10
Cheyne, George 45
child-bed fever 34
child mortality 17
childbirth 17, 45
cholera 25, 35, 85
Christian hospitals 66
church, role of 30, 56, 64-5

circulation of the blood 58
Clean Air Acts 90
cleanliness 13
computed tomography (CT) 61
Coventry 81
Crimean War 71, 73
CT (computed tomography) 61
Culpepper, Nicholas 45
Curie, Marie 49, 118

Davy, Sir Humphrey 46
Dee, John 32
DNA (deoxyribonucleic acid) 62

early modern period, treatments 44-5
eating, healthy 92
Edward I 16
Ehrlich, Paul 59
eighteenth century
    disease prevention 34-7
    hospitals 68-9
endowed hospitals 68-9
Eyam, Derbyshire 94, 98-105

famine 15
Farr, William 84
fitness drives 92
Fleming, Alexander 50
Florey, Howard 50
Floyer, Sir John 45
flu pandemic 26
four humours 8, 17, 30, 43, 55
frostbite 112

Galen 55, 57
gas attacks 111
genetic engineering 62
Gerard of York 32
germ theory 9, 40, 59
God, and disease 9, 17, 30
Gordon, Alexander 34
Great Plague 96-105

Harvey, William 58
healthy lifestyles 91-2
healthy living pyramid 12
height 11
herbal medicine 8, 42, 45
Hippocrates 8, 30, 55
holistic medicine 52
homeopathy 52
hospitals 65-70
housing 89-90
Housing Act (1919) 89
Human Genome Project 62
hygiene 18-21

immunisation 36-9
industrialisation 24-5, 68, 83
infant mortality rate 38
infection 112, 117
inoculation 36

Jenner, Edward 36-7

Koch, Robert 40, 48, 59

leeches 43, 44
leper hospitals 65
Liberal reforms 74, 75-6
lice 112
life expectancy 11
Lind, James 35
Lister, Joseph 47
Liston, Robert 9, 46
Lloyd George, David 75

magnetic resonance imaging (MRI) 61
major offensives, Western Front 110
malnutrition 14-15, 24
medieval era
    causes of illness 14-21
    doctors 33
    medical ideas 54
    patient care 64-6
    public health 80-1
    treatments 42-4
mental illness 45
midwifery 45
MMR vaccine 39
mortality bill 22
Mother Shipton 33
MRI (magnetic resonance imaging) 61

National Insurance Acts (1911/13) 75
new towns 90
NHS (National Health Service) 76-8
Nightingale, Florence 71-2
nineteenth century
    medical knowledge 59
    patient care 70
    public health 83-8
nursing 71-3, 115

Paré, Ambroise 57
Pasteur, Louis 9, 40, 59
patient care
    eighteenth century 68-9
    medieval era to mid-sixteenth century 64-6
    nineteenth century 70
    voluntary charities 67
penicillin 8, 50

PET (positron emission tomography) 61
plague 23, 94–7
    see also Eyam, Derbyshire
plastic surgery 116
pneumonic plague 94
positron emission tomography (PET) 61
poverty 14, 89
prevention of illness and disease
    early methods 30–3
    eighteenth century 34–7
public health
    medieval era 80–1
    NHS 9
    nineteenth century 83–8
    seventeenth century 82
    sixteenth century 82
    twentieth century 89–90
    twenty-first century 91–2
Public Health Act 85

quarantine 98–105

radiation 49, 51
RAMC (Royal Army Medical Corps) 115
rat fleas 95
Reeves, Maud Pember 89
Renaissance 57
rickets 24
Röntgen, Wilhelm 60
Rowntree, Seebohm 89
Royal Army Medical Corps (RAMC) 115
royal hospitals 67
Royal Societies 68

Salt, Titus 86–7
scanning techniques 60–1
school meals 74
scientific method 35

scurvy 35
Seacole, Mary 73
Semmelweis, Ignaz 34, 47
seventeenth century
    illnesses 22–3
    medical knowledge 57–8
    public health 82
Sharp, Jane 45
shell shock 112
Simpson, James 46
sixteenth century
    medical knowledge 57
    patient care 64–6
    public health 82
slum clearance 90
smallpox 36–7
smog 90
Snow, John 35
soothsayers 33
Southwood Smith, Thomas 84
St John, Lady Johanna 45
supernatural 17
surgery
    transplant 51
    without anaesthetics 9
surgical clothing 48

Thomas splints 117
town life 20, 24–5
transplant surgery 51
treatments
    early modern period 44–5
    medieval era 42–4
    twentieth century 49–52
trench fever 112
trench foot 112, 113
trench warfare 107–10
twentieth century
    diseases 26–8
    medical knowledge 60–2
    public health 89–90
    treatments 49–52
twenty-first century, public health 91–2
typhoid 25

ultrasound 61
urine 43

vaccination 36–9, 116
Vesalius, Andreas 57
Victorian era 24–5
viral infections 27–8
voluntary charities, hospitals 67

warfare 16, 107–10
waste disposal 80–1
water 9, 13, 20, 34
Welfare State 74, 76–8
Western Front
    casualties 114–15
    disease 112–13
    illness 112–13
    injuries 111–12
    major offensives 110
    medical advances 116–19
    treatment of wounded 114–15
    trench warfare 107–10
    wounds 111–12
William the Conqueror 15
Withering, William 45
World War I 107–19
    see also Western Front

X-rays 60, 118

zodiac chart 43

Acknowledgements

The Publishers would like to thank the following for permission to reproduce copyright material.

Photos credits
p. 7t © Jochen Sands/DigitalVision/Thinkstock/Getty Images; p. 7m © Justin Kase zsixz/Alamy Stock Photo; p. 7b ©Martin Siepmann/Stockbyte/Getty Images; p. 10 © Georgios Kollidas/iStock/Getty Images; p. 12 © Okea/iStock/Thinkstock; p. 16 © The British Library Board (Royal 20 C. VII, f.51); p. 20 The Black Death (gouache on paper), Nicolle, Pat (Patrick) (1907–95)/Private Collection/© Look and Learn/Bridgeman Images; p. 22 ©Wellcome Images (available under Creative Commons Attribution only licence CC BY 4.0); p. 23 © INTERFOTO/Alamy Stock Photo; p. 24 ©Wellcome Images (available under Creative Commons Attribution only licence CC BY 4.0); p. 25l © Mary Evans Picture Library/Alamy Stock Photo; p. 25r © Maidstone Museum & Bentlif Art Gallery; p. 26 © Jean Williamson/Alamy Stock Photo; p. 27 ©The National Library of Medicine; p. 30 © Niday Picture Library/Alamy Stock Photo; p. 31 © Heritage Image Partnership Ltd/Alamy Stock Photo; p. 32 © classicpaintings/Alamy Stock Photo; p. 33 © Mary Evans Picture Library/Alamy Stock Photo; p. 34 ©Wellcome Images (available under Creative Commons Attribution only licence CC BY 4.0); p. 35 © The Granger Collection/TopFoto; p. 37 ©Wellcome Images (available under Creative Commons Attribution only licence CC BY 4.0); p. 40l ©Wellcome Images (available under Creative Commons Attribution only licence CC BY 4.0); p. 40r ©Wellcome Images (available under Creative Commons Attribution only licence CC BY 4.0); p. 43t © Robana/Rex/Shutterstock; p. 43m ©Wellcome Images (available under Creative Commons Attribution only licence CC BY 4.0); p. 43b ©Wellcome Images (available under Creative Commons Attribution only licence CC BY 4.0); p. 44r ©The Art Archive/Alamy Stock Photo; p. 44l © age fotostock/Alamy Stock Photo; p. 46l ©Wellcome Images (available under Creative Commons Attribution only licence CC BY 4.0); p. 46r ©Wellcome Images (available under Creative Commons Attribution only licence CC BY 4.0); p. 47 ©Wellcome Images (available under Creative Commons Attribution only licence CC BY 4.0); p. 49 © World History Archive/Alamy Stock Photo; p. 50 © Science and Society/Superstock; p. 56 ©Wellcome Images (available under Creative Commons Attribution only licence CC BY 4.0); p. 58 ©Wellcome Images (available under Creative Commons Attribution only licence CC BY 4.0); p. 60t © Universal History Archive/Getty Images; p. 60b © Old Visuals/Alamy Stock Photo; p. 61 © Westend61 GmbH/Alamy Stock Photo; p. 62 © Science Photo Library/Alamy Stock Photo; p. 69 © Heritage Image Partnership Ltd/Alamy Stock Photo; p. 71l ©Wellcome Images (available under Creative Commons Attribution only licence CC BY 4.0); p. 71r ©Wellcome Images (available under Creative Commons Attribution only licence CC BY 4.0); p. 72 ©Wellcome Images (available under Creative Commons Attribution only licence CC BY 4.0); p. 73l © Amoret Tanner/Alamy Stock Photo; p. 73r Supplied by Llyfrgell Genedlaethol Cymru/National Library of Wales; p. 74 © The National Archives, London. England/Mary Evans.; p. 75 Trades Union Congress Library Collections, London Metropolitan University; p. 76 © Pictorial Press Ltd/Alamy Stock Photo; p. 78 © Mirrorpix; p. 80 courtesy of John D Clare; p. 81 © North Wind Picture Archives/Alamy Stock Photo; p. 82 © London Metropolitan Archives; p. 83 © The Granger Collection/TopFoto; p. 84 © SSPL/Getty Images); p. 85 © The National Archives; p. 86 © Mary Evans Picture Library/Alamy Stock Photo; p. 87 © Pictorial Press Ltd/Alamy Stock Photo; p. 88 © Hulton Archive/Getty Images; p. 90 © RDImages/Epics/Getty Images; p. 92 © Public Health England; p. 94 © INTERFOTO/Alamy Stock Photo; p. 95l © NIAID; p. 95r © blickwinkel/Alamy Stock Photo; p. 97 © V&A Images/Alamy Stock Photo; p. 99 © David Lyons/Alamy Stock Photo; p. 100t William Mompesson, Rector of Eyam (oil on panel), English School, (17th century)/© Sheffield Galleries and Museums Trust, UK/Bridgeman Images; p. 100b © Philip Jones/Alamy Stock Photo; p. 101 © WilliamRobinson/Alamy Stock Photo; p. 102 © travelib/Alamy Stock Photo; p. 105 © Rick Edwards/Alamy Stock Photo; p. 111 © Pictorial Press Ltd/Alamy Stock Photo; p. 113t © Chronicle/Alamy Stock Photo; p. 113b © Trustees of the Army Medical Services Museum/Wellcome Images; p. 114 © World History Archive/TopFoto; p. 116 © Chronicle/Alamy Stock Photo; p. 121tl © Bettmann/Contributor/Getty Images; p. 121b © Davies/Getty Images; p. 121tr © Media Minds/Alamy Stock Photo; p. 122tl courtesy of John D Clare; p. 122b © RDImages/Epics/Getty Images; p. 122tr © The National Archives; p. 123 ©Wellcome Images (available under Creative Commons Attribution only licence CC BY 4.0); p. 124 ©Wellcome Images (available under Creative Commons Attribution only licence CC BY 4.0).

Text acknowledgements
p. 15 From *The Anglo-Saxon Chronicle*, from Terry Jones and Alan Ereira Medieval Lives, BBC Books, page 29. Copyright © by Random House Publishing Group; p. 39 Copyright Guardian News & Media Ltd 2016; p. 42 The Knight With the Lion, written by Helen Lynch and designed by Helen Lynch and Susan Dunbar ©1996 The University of Aberdeen; p. 48 From The Greatest Benefit to Mankind by Roy Porter (Fontana Press, 1999), p. 373; p. 49 From Mme. Curie is Dead; Martyr To Science, New York Times, 1934. URL: http://www.nytimes.com/learning/general/onthisday/bday/1107.html?pagewanted=all; p. 62 © Carl Engelking/Discover Magazine; p. 91 © Telegraph Media Group Limited 2015; p. 109 From *Schools History Project* (2009) by Dale Banham and Ian Luff; p. 102 A Book of Golden Deeds By Charlotte M. Yonge (1864); p. 111 S. Millard, I Saw Them Die: Diary and Recollections of Shirley Millard (1936, Houghton Mifflin Harcourt); **Table 8.3, p. 115** © Crown Copyright; p. 117 Surgeon-General Sir Anthony Bowlby, *The Development of British Surgery at the Front*, British Medical Journal, 1917; 1:705; p. 118 THE ROSES OF NO MAN'S LAND by Lyn Macdonald (Michael Joseph 1980, Penguin Books 1993). Copyright © Lyn Macdonald, 1980.